Alcohol, Cocaine, and Accidents

Drug and Alcohol Abuse Reviews

Edited by

Ronald R. Watson

Drug and Alcohol Abuse Reviews • 7

Alcohol, Cocaine, and Accidents

Edited by

Ronald R. Watson

University of Arizona, Tucson, Arizona

Humana Press • Totowa, New Jersey

Printed in the United States of America. 9 8 7 6 5 4 3 2 1

Library of Congress Cataloging-in-Publication Data

Alcohol, cocaine, and accidents/edited by Ronald R. Watson.
    p. cm.—(Drug and alcohol abuse reviews; 7)
  Includes index.
  ISBN 0-89603-294-9
  1. Drinking and traffic accidents. 2. Automobile drivers—Drug abuse.
3. Cocaine habit. 4. Alcoholism—Prevention. 5. Cocaine habit—Prevention.
I. Watson, Ronald R. (Ronald Ross)   II. Series.
HE5620.DA6255 1995
363.12'51—dc20   94-45440
                                              CIP

Contents

Preface

Alcohol is involved in more than 100,000 premature deaths in the United States each year, with a significant number of such deaths involving accidents of various types. Drinking clearly increases the risk of injury and death, depending on the activity or situation. Thus, strategies designed to prevent or reduce the risk of alcohol-related traumas are best directed at drinking patterns or settings that involve significant risk.

Young people's attitudes and behaviors toward drinking and driving have been demonstrated to have significant effects on risk of injury or accident. Similarly, aquatic injuries are highly associated with the use of alcohol. Aviation safety, especially of noncommercial planes, already requires the absence of alcohol use.

An understanding of how alcohol increases the risk of injury is the key to preventing or reducing risky behavior. Intervention programs designed to prevent alcohol-related accidents include community prevention, as well as treatment to reduce alcohol's modification of physiological function and the attendant trauma. Thus, by understanding the nature of alcohol's involvement in risky behaviors and accidents, strategies to reduce them can more readily be developed. Cocaine, which recently has been implicated in an increasing number of injuries, is also reviewed. This is important because the use in our society of a variety of drugs of abuse that alter the central nervous system is currently increasing.

Alcohol, Cocaine, and Accidents is the first book to bring together key critical reviews of the effects of alcohol and cocaine on accident causation, and offers what we believe are effective strategies and programs designed to bring risky consumption under optimal control.

Ronald R. Watson

Contributors

Nicole Bell • *Social and Behavioral Sciences Department, Boston University School of Public Health, Boston, MA*

Richard H. Blake • *Counseling Department, University of Nebraska at Omaha, Omaha, NE*

Mary-Ellen Fortini • *Occupational Health Services Corporation, Larkspur, CA*

Joel W. Grube • *Prevention Research Center, Berkeley, CA*

Paul J. Gruenewald • *Prevention Research Center, Berkeley, CA*

Wayne Harrison • *Counseling Department, University of Nebraska at Omaha, Omaha, NE*

Ralph Hingson • *Social and Behavioral Sciences Department, Boston University School of Public Health, Boston, MA*

Harold D. Holder • *Prevention Research Center, Berkeley, CA*

Jonathan Howland • *Social and Behavioral Sciences Department, Boston University School of Public Health, Boston, MA*

David P. MacKinnon • *Department of Psychology, Arizona State University, Tempe, AZ*

Thomas Mangione • *Social and Behavioral Sciences Department, Boston University School of Public Health, Boston, MA*

Peter Marzuk • *Department of Psychiatry, Cornell University Medical College, New York*

Carol Lederhaus Popkin • *Occupational Health Services Corporation, Larkspur, CA*

Leonard E. Ross • *Center for Aviation and Aerospace Research, Embry-Riddle Aeronautical University, Daytona Beach, FL*

Susan M. Ross • *Center for Aviation and Aerospace Research, Embry-Riddle Aeronautical University, Daytona Beach, FL*

Robert F. Saltz • *Prevention Research Center, Berkeley, CA*

Gordon Smith • *Social and Behavioral Sciences Department, Boston University School of Public Health, Boston, MA*

Kenneth Tardiff • *Department of Psychiatry, Section on Epidemiology and Community Psychiatry, Cornell University Medical College, New York*

Andrew J. Treno • *Prevention Research Center, Berkeley, CA*

Robert B. Voas • *Prevention Research Center, Berkeley, CA*

William F. Wieczorek • *Research Institute on Addictions, Buffalo, NY*

Identification
of Aging Adults
with Alcohol Problems

Richard H. Blake and Wayne Harrison

Introduction

Even without the potential impact of alcohol use, aging is associated with numerous changes that put the elderly at increased risk for accidents. Changes in vision, hearing, coordination, strength, and flexibility are only a few examples. Many health conditions, such as diabetes and heart disease, and the comparatively heavy use of medications,[1,2] are all factors placing the elderly in special jeopardy from alcohol use.

Intoxication or alcohol-induced effects such as drowsiness can lead to mistakes in taking medications. Alcohol alters the effectiveness of many medications commonly taken by older persons, and may lead to toxic effects. Physicians unaware of their patients' alcohol use can misdiagnose conditions that are masked by alcohol. Patients can be, and are, prescribed medications without their physicians having sufficient knowledge of their alcohol use to safely prescribe the medication.[3]

Not only are the elderly at heightened risk for a wide variety of accidents, they are susceptible to increasingly severe consequences from accidents. A fall that may result in embarrassment or a bruise in a younger person may lead to broken bones, surgery, extended rehabilitation, and a range of medical complications and permanently diminished function in an older person.

From: *Drug and Alcohol Abuse Reviews, Vol. 7: Alcohol, Cocaine, and Accidents*
Ed.: R. R. Watson ©1995 Humana Press Inc., Totowa, NJ

To our knowledge, there is no instrument for screening older persons whose drinking behavior identifies them specifically for risk of accidents. There are, however, numerous procedures and instruments for identifying persons whose use of alcohol is associated with adverse consequences, suggestive of an added risk of accidents. For the most part, these procedures and instruments reflect an emphasis on alcoholism or alcohol dependence, rather than a broader conception of hazardous or problem drinking and they are not specific to older persons. Readers interested in general issues pertaining to alcohol screening, assessment, or diagnosis are referred to available reviews.[4-10]

In this chapter we consider some of the factors that may complicate identification of older problem drinkers, discuss two of the most used questionnaires for identifying alcoholics, and describe two new screening questionnaires specifically for use with older people. One of these, the Problem Drinking Screen for Seniors (PDSS), which we have developed, is described in some detail.

Problems in Identifying Older Problem Drinkers

It is widely suggested that there are special obstacles to the detection of older problem drinkers that result in underidentification.[11-17] The suggested reasons for this special difficulty are briefly discussed.

Differences in Life Status

Differences in employment, family, and health status may decrease the likelihood of problem drinking being identified. Retirement, for example, can mean a reduced contact with others and a reduction in observable performance requirements that permits drinking to go unrecognized.[15,17-19] Increased likelihood of widowhood, living alone, and a general reduction in the social network and such activities as driving are also possible obstacles to identification.[15,17,19,20]

Indicators of alcohol problems, even if observed by relatives or others, may be misunderstood or discounted. Many of the behaviors or changes that might raise suspicion of alcohol problems in a younger person may, with an elderly person, be attributed to health conditions or mistaken notions of normal aging. Confusion, memory lapses, sleep disturbance, depression, or other affective changes, accidents, and tremors are examples of problem signs that can easily be misinterpreted.[21]

Similarly, many of the laboratory tests used in identifying alcohol abusers are not highly specific to alcohol use with the elderly. As examples, liver function abnormalities, anemia, vitamin deficiencies, platelet disorders, bleeding abnormalities, and hyperuricemia can result from either alcohol use or from other medical problems commonly encountered in the elderly.[21-24]

Difficulties with Basic Alcohol Assessment Domains

Important questions have been raised regarding the suitability for older people of basic concepts and domains typically included in alcohol questionnaires and diagnoses.[13,19,25,26]

In a frequently cited article, Graham[13] identified specific weaknesses in the application of five common alcohol assessment domains to older persons (social consequences, health problems, self-report of quantity and frequency, symptoms of drunkenness and dependence, and self-recognition of problem). Some of her criticisms reflect aspects of life circumstances previously mentioned. As examples, in the social consequences domain, questionnaire items pertaining to work-related difficulties or troubles with spouse may be less appropriate because of lessened work role and increased likelihood of being single. Graham suggested that the elderly may be less able to recognize their own problems because of decreased social contact and fewer obligations and the resulting reduction in feedback from others and their own experience. The elderly may also misinterpret alcohol problems as health problems. Thus, questions requiring self-identification may be of reduced effectiveness. Alcohol questionnaire items in the health problems domain may also be less useful simply because of the increased incidence of health problems associated with aging.

Another suggested weakness of questionnaire items is the possible inability of older people to respond properly to items requiring accurate memory of past consumption (e.g., How much did you drink last week?) or calculating ability (e.g., What is your usual consumption?).

Also suspect is the willingness of older persons to respond honestly to alcohol-related questions. It is suggested that denial is particularly likely among the elderly. There is also a question of what cutoff levels to set when using alcohol consumption criteria. Because the physical response to alcohol differs with age, it is doubtful that the same cutoffs should apply for determining problem or heavy drinking.

Items representing the dependence domain are also thought to be problematic because they are likely to be based on inaccurate self-report and are susceptible to having dependence symptoms confounded with symptoms of aging. Graham considered items in this domain, which reflect severe and obvious indications, such as withdrawal symptoms, to be especially likely to engender denial among those not already in treatment programs.

The *DSM–III–R*[27] diagnostic criteria are not excluded from similar criticisms. Atkinson[12] specifically questioned the appropriateness for older persons of three criteria used in *DSM–III–R* (time spent in dependence-related behaviors, role interference caused by dependence, and reduction of normal activities caused by dependence). Extrapolating from data obtained with the Alcohol Stages Index (ASI) on older persons whose driving licenses had been revoked for driving while intoxicated, Mulford and Fitzgerald[28] suggested that over half of these known problem drinkers would probably not meet the *DSM–III–R* or most other clinical alcoholism diagnostic criteria.

Attitudes of Erstwhile Identifiers

Willenbring and Spring[29] suggested that "Of the various factors that affect screening and diagnosis of drinking problems, our feelings and beliefs about drinking and drunks are arguably the most important" (p. 27). They consider educational, personal, and cultural factors all to be working against proper evaluation and care of older problem drinkers. Abrams and Alexopoulos[18] suggested that there is probably an insidious age bias where physicians are involved, which reflects that of the larger society. They pointed out that age itself has been identified as a risk factor for inadequate treatment by health care personnel. Others[17,30] have also expressed concern that identification of elderly problem drinkers is hampered by social stereotypes and professional bias.

Concerns regarding bias are supported by research, two examples being Curtis et al.[24] and Moos et al.[31] The former found that hospital physicians identified a substantially smaller proportion of older persons who had been independently screened positive for alcoholism than younger persons who had been so screened (37 vs 60%). Even when diagnosed, the elderly alcoholics were less likely to be recommended for treatment. Further, Curtis et al. found that when recommended for treatment, the elderly were less likely to be given treatment. Moos et al. found a similar pattern with Veterans Administration patients with respect to differences in treatment rates by age. They also found that treatment, when given, was more likely to be oriented toward medical management for the elderly, and more rehabilitative for the younger patients. Such findings suggest more than technical difficulties in screening; they imply age bias.

Second Thoughts
on Special Identification Problems

Although accepting the general legitimacy of the concerns identified regarding differences in life status, alcohol assessment domains, and attitudes of erstwhile identifiers, it is possible that some of the underlying considerations may not be quite so negative or clear, as has been suspected. Consider the following examples.

Marital Rates

A substantial gender difference exists with respect to marital status among the elderly. A much larger proportion of older men are married than are women. Hayward and Liu[32] reported marital rates of 75 and 82% for women and men, respectively, at ages 50–54; 55 and 83%, respectively, at ages 65–69; and 43 and 79%, respectively, at ages 70–74. It is true that the proportion of single people increases with age, but caution is warranted in interpreting such information. Overgeneralizing can be misleading. Although widowhood may result in a reduction in the number of potential identifiers of problem drinking, this is only a possible reduction. It is also possible that children or others may intensify their contact with the widowed senior. Or, the widowed person may move in with someone else, or into a residence center where regular and meaningful contact with others may actually increase. It is also possible for a spouse to be an enabler for problematic drinking and to be an obstacle, rather than an aid, in identification. The loss of a spouse may make long-needed identification and treatment a more likely occurrence for the survivor.

Inability to Remember

The concern that older persons may be relatively unable to respond to questions requiring memory or mental calculations, and may thus not have the ability to provide information, may be excessive.[33] The extent of impaired memory function is not substantial in most older persons. From their review of research on memory, learning, and attention in aging, Sugar and McDowd[34] concluded that "...from a practical point of view, observed differences due to age may be insignificant, though theoretically interesting" (p. 310). Furthermore, the magnitudes of age-related differences reported in the research literature over the last three decades seem to have shrunk.[35] In the absence of pathology, the vast majority of older people function amply well to meet the requirements of completing most alcohol questionnaires.

The incidence of pathology sufficient to interfere with performance on such instruments is very low among noninstitutionalized elderly. Survey-based estimates for prevalence of moderate and severe dementia in elderly populations generally range "upward from about 1%, centering close to 5% and with almost all values falling between 2 and 14%" (p. 33).[36] The likelihood of difficulty increases with age, but there is probably no age at which most people are so cognitively impaired as to be unable to respond informatively regarding their drinking. Even when older persons claim poor memory, their self-assessment is very likely wrong.[37]

Because heavy, sustained use of alcohol is itself a cause of cognitive disorders, and some older persons do have cognitive dysfunction as well as depression that can affect functional memory, it is not unusual to find older persons in alcohol treatment who will be unable to answer questions accurately. This can make assessment and diagnosis more difficult. Nevertheless, this is the exception, not the norm, and especially so among the general population of noninstitutionalized older drinkers. Furthermore, effective and efficient means are available for screening for cognitive problems where it appears appropriate to do so.[38–40]

In our view, the inability of older persons to provide information about their drinking is less likely to be a problem than mistaken beliefs and attitudes among relatives, physicians, or others who may be potential case finders. The belief that cognitive dysfunction is normal or prevalent for older persons, for example, can discourage testing for alcohol misuse, and reduce the likelihood of accurate or timely identification of the true problem.

Denial

Related to the concern that older persons may not be able to respond accurately to alcohol questions is the suspicion that problem drinkers tend to deny or minimize their drinking or resulting negative consequences.[6,41] Special doubts in this regard have been directed toward the elderly.

The considerable research on the validity of self-reports has been reviewed elsewhere.[42–44] Babor et al.[42] found that all concurrent validation studies using the agreement of collateral informants with the drinker's self-reporting as the criterion showed "moderate-to-good statistically significant, positive correlations" (p. 415). Other reviewers have reached essentially similar conclusions. As an example, O'Farrell and Maiston[44] stated "clinical lore and the empirical literature on alcoholics' self-referral are in marked contrast to each other. The skepticism of alcoholics' self-reports that remains in the alcohol field seems to come, at least in part, from an overgeneralization from clinical and everyday experiences with alcoholics to their behavior in a treatment outcome assessment context" (p. 103). Studies reported since these reviews,[5,45–51] including one specific to adults over age 60,[52] tend to support these general positive conclusions regarding the efficacy of self-reports on alcohol use and problems.

Self-reports are widely used and have been studied in many fields, including gerontology.[53–58] In a study comparing the quality of self-report data among older and younger chronically ill patients, Sherbourne and Meredith[56] found some significant differences but their conclusion was that "self-report health data can be gathered from older patients as well as younger patients without significant decrements in data quality...we found that declines in reliability with age are very small" (p. 5209). Studies ranging from self-reports of bowel symptoms to sexual problems find self-reports of older people to be essentially valid and useful. This at least should not discourage the use of self-reporting methods with older people as a way of identifying alcohol use and problems.

The evidence seems strong that under certain conditions individuals are able and willing to give accurate reports of many personal behaviors and conditions, including alcohol use. It has been suggested[42] that the important issue is no longer whether self-report data are valid but rather how such data can be made more valid. It is clear that the types of questions, the time lag involved, and other factors can impact the validity of self-reports. Of particular importance for interpreting research evidence regarding denial is the difference between data collection for research and for clinical screening purposes. In research, subjects can be assured of confidentiality and freed of what might be seen as adverse consequences of being honest (e.g., confronted or forced into treatment). The validity of self-reports has been less well established in clinical screening where possible intervention based on client responses is the reality. Studies of self-report validity based on persons already in treatment or assured of confidentiality do not directly address the validity of self-reports for identifying older problem drinkers for screening purposes. Neither do studies of self-report validity conducted on younger persons. Nevertheless, research results are encouraging, and the number of older people not asked about their drinking when they should be asked is surely a larger number than those who falsify or lie when asked.

Use of Selected Alcohol Screening Questionnaires with Older Persons

Two of the most widely used screening questionnaires for identifying alcoholics are the CAGE[59] and the Michigan Alcoholism Screening Test (MAST).[60] Though neither was developed on nor intended specifically for use with older persons, recent studies of these questionnaires have begun to provide evidence regarding their utility with older persons. We discuss this evidence in the following sections. We are aware of two additional screening questionnaires that were developed specifically for use with older persons. One of these, the Michigan Alcoholism Screening Test–Geriatric Version (MAST–G),[61] is also discussed at this point. We report the development of the other, the PDSS, in a subsequent section.

CAGE

The CAGE screening questionnaire[59,62] consists of four questions:

1. Have you ever felt you should cut down on your drinking?
2. Have people annoyed you by criticizing your drinking?
3. Have you ever felt bad or guilty about your drinking?
4. Have you ever had a drink first thing in the morning to steady your nerves or get rid of a hangover (eye-opener)?

CAGE is an acronym for key words or phrases in the four questions: cut down, annoyed, guilty, eye-opener.

Although several studies not specific to the elderly have supported the CAGE,[63-67] others have not, or at least have suggested limitations.[46,68-70] Waterson and Murray-Lyon[71] expressed concerns and cited evidence regarding the continued validity of two CAGE questions (questions 1 and 3). Their concern was based on the impact of broad public education efforts regarding potential dangers of alcohol use that they suggested could lead people to express more guilt or thoughts of cutting down in relation to drinking level. Waterson and Murray-Lyon were addressing a British readership and made reference to particular alcohol education efforts in Great Britain, but their concern, if valid, could be equally applicable to other countries or areas where similar educational efforts and attitudinal changes exist. Response patterns to CAGE questions may be changing in ways that alter validity. None of the aforementioned studies were specific to identifying older problem drinkers, and they vary in design and completeness of reporting.

Buchsbaum et al.[72] assessed CAGE performance with persons age 60 or over as part of a larger study. Three hundred twenty-three elderly patients at an ambulatory medical clinic served as subjects. All subjects were assured of confidentiality. The alcohol module of the Diagnostic Interview Schedule (DIS)[73] was used to classify respondents. Patients were defined as alcohol abusers or dependent if they met the *DSM-III*[74] criteria for these disorders, as assessed with the DIS. Patients who reported at least one symptom on the DIS, but did not meet *DSM-III* criteria for abuse or dependence, were categorized as problem drinkers. Dependent, abuser, and problem drinkers combined ($n = 106$) constituted about one-third of the total of 323 patients. Using a CAGE score of 2 or higher (often considered the standard for identifying alcoholics) the observed sensitivity (proportion of positive cases correctly identified) was .698, specificity (proportion of negative cases correctly identified) was .908, and the positive predictive value was .787. Using a CAGE score of 1 or higher, sensitivity was .858, specificity was

.780, and the positive predictive value was .659. Subjects were also divided for analysis according to the recency of symptoms reported. Patients were considered active if they reported the most recent symptom had occurred within 1 yr of testing, and in remission if the most recent symptom occurred prior to 1 yr of testing. Of the 106 patients who met the criteria of abuse, dependence, or problem drinking, 18 reported their problem was active and 88 were in remission. The lifetime prevalence for drinking problems was 63% for men and 27% for women.

MAST

The MAST is a 25-item questionnaire listing various signs and symptoms of alcoholism. Persons completing the questionnaire are asked if the signs or symptoms have ever applied to them ("yes" or "no"), and, in some instances, how many times an event has occurred. There are different ways in which the MAST can be scored, as well as shorter versions of the questionnaire, the Brief MAST (BMAST) with 10 items,[75] and the Short MAST (SMAST) with 13 items.[76] There are other variations and readers are referred to the several reviews and descriptions that are available.[6,77–82]

Willenbring et al.[83] examined the validity of the MAST, BMAST, and SMAST with men age 60 or older. Two scoring methods were used with the MAST. Weighted scoring assigns different values to different items. Unit scoring assigns equal value to each positive answer. A sample of 52 hospitalized alcoholics and 33 nonalcoholics, mostly hospital patients, was used. Alcoholic subjects were consecutive admissions to a single alcohol/drug dependency treatment program and met the criteria for alcohol abuse or dependence of the *DSM–III*. The nonalcoholic controls were screened on multiple criteria intended to determine alcoholism.

All versions of the MAST discriminated well between alcoholics and controls. Depending on cutoff scores used, sensitivity was reported as ranging from .82–1.00, and specificity from .72–1.00. Using a cutoff score of 5+, the weighted-scored MAST had a sensitivity of 1.00 and a specificity of .83. The unit-scored MAST had a sensitivity of .96 and a specificity of .86 using a cutoff score of 3+. The BMAST had a sensitivity of .91 and a specificity of .83 using a 4+ score. The SMAST had sensitivity and specificity of .98 and .72, respectively, using a 2+ score. Factor analysis of the Brief and Short versions suggested a factor structure similar to that which has been found previously with younger subjects. Findings were interpreted as supporting the validity of the MAST with older men; Willenbring et al. particularly recommended the unit-scored MAST or SMAST for screening because of their performance and ease of scoring. Elsewhere, Willenbring and Spring[29] emphasized that the MAST will screen for alcoholism but not for medically hazardous drinking that must be assessed using measures of alcohol use.[83]

Yersin et al.[84] reported a MAST validation study in which subjects, age 20–75 yr, were divided into age groups for data analysis. This study attempted to assess the feasibility of using the French translation of the MAST with a French-speaking population in Switzerland. A clinical diagnosis of alcoholism was used as the criterion. The exact procedure used by the clinicians in making the diagnosis is not clear, although it apparently included "biological abnormalities," "anamnestic," and other "clinical" factors (p. 2071). Results were reported in predictive values. For the 53 subjects age 50–59 yr, the predictive value was .67 for a MAST score of 5+ and .89 for a score of 4 or less. For the 137 subjects age 60–75, the predictive value was .61 for a score of 5+ and .92 for a score of 4 or less. Kappa coefficients of agreement according to critical MAST score and diagnosis were .57 for the 50–59 age group and .51 for the 60–67 age group. By comparison, Kappa coefficients for young persons were higher, .77 for age 20–39 and .71 for age 40–49.

In a study attempting to evaluate a screening procedure for chemical abuse among persons age 65 and over,[85] it was found that the BMAST could be eliminated from the screening procedure without loss of case identification. Also, a correlation of .407 was found between the BMAST and CAGE in these older patients.

Other studies of MAST validity have included older persons as part of the total group of subjects but have not reported performance information separately for the older subjects. Generally, the MAST showed a good ability to identify alcoholics in these mixed-age studies.[86,87]

MAST–G

The MAST–G consists of 24 items; respondents are to respond "yes" or "no" to each item. Some of the items are not stated with a specified time frame (e.g., "Does having a drink help you sleep?"), but clearly imply a current time perspective. Other items are presented with an "ever" or lifelong perspective. Scoring is a simple unit system and consists of summing the "yes" responses, with 5 or more "yes" responses "indicative of alcohol problem." Development of the MAST–G started from a pool of 94 trial items that were reduced in two stages using 840 and 305 elderly subjects for testing. A diagnosis of alcohol dependence *(DSM–III–R)* was used as the validation standard. Blow et al.[61] reported a sensitivity of 93.9% and a specificity of 78.1% with a positive predictive value of 87.2% and negative predictive value of 88.9%. It is also reported that factor analysis identified five underlying symptom domains and that other research has demonstrated that the MAST–G performs better with older persons than either the original MAST or the CAGE.

PDSS

Research Objectives

The two principle objectives of the present research were the development of a screening instrument for identifying older problem drinkers and a cross-validation assessment of this instrument. Included in the cross-validation were tests of the discriminating ability of the instrument and a validity comparison with existing screening measures. Development of the PDSS was guided by the following goals:

1. Inclusion of older adult-specific problem domains;
2. Use of questionnaire items that were not offensive or irrelevant to older adults;
3. A focus on recent behavior and problems;
4. A response format that permitted a degree of respondent denial without nullifying screening effectiveness;
5. Ease of administration and scoring; and
6. Psychometric properties superior to existing instruments.

To obtain an unbiased assessment of the screening instrument's validity, the development of the instrument and the estimation of its validity were undertaken as separate phases of the research.

Method

Item Development

An initial pool of approximately 500 items was established, representing four primary domains:

1. Consumption (quantity, frequency, history, time, place, and occasion of use);
2. Dependence symptoms (withdrawal, tolerance, and psychological dependence);
3. Negative consequences (negative physical and psychological effects, perceived negative impact on life circumstances, and concerns about drinking); and
4. Benefits (general positive cognitions antecedent to drinking).

Successive drafts of items were developed based on information gained from judges with experience in working with older persons, from consultants having expertise in alcohol screening, and from a series of trial administrations. A total of 48 persons age 60 or over participated in the trial administrations.

Items were selected for continued use on the basis of representative-ness of selected domains, the responses and comments made by the pilot subjects, and observations made by those who administered the question-naires. Final selection of items was reached by consensus of the researchers and consultants. This first phase concluded with agreement on a set of 131 items.

In the next phase 373 interviews were completed. On the basis of analy-ses of these data, 34 items were retained as a screening instrument. This instrument, three health-related items, and seven items pertaining to amount and pattern of consumption were employed in a cross-validation study. Sub-jects were also given the CAGE and the MAST questionnaires.

Subjects

Two categories of subjects were included in this research: an alcohol treatment group and persons who were not in a treatment program. The alcohol treatment group consisted of males and females age 50 or over cur-rently in one of 14 treatment programs. Individuals who were abusing other drugs or had dual diagnoses were included if the treatment program had determined alcohol as the primary drug of use. All subjects were paid for their participation with the exception of those in one program. Refusals to participate were rare (<3%).

The nontreatment group comprised noninstitutionalized persons age 50 or over who were paid volunteer participants. Their participation was solicited through senior volunteer programs, veterans and service organiza-tions, senior centers, and senior residence facilities. A criterion for eligibil-ity was consumption of at least one alcoholic beverage in the preceding year; this criterion was raised to one drink on at least five occasions during the preceding year for the cross-validation study.

A total of 837 seniors participated in the study: 48 in the first phase, 373 in the second phase, and 416 in the cross-validation study. Demographic characteristics of the cross-validation sample are reported in Table 1.

Data Collection

All data were collected from individual subjects by a trained interviewer after obtaining written informed consent and demographic information. Any participant whose cognitive ability to respond to the questionnaire was suspect was also administered the Short Portable Mental Status Questionnaire.[40] Less than 1% of individuals interviewed were eliminated from further participation on this basis. Interviews of nontreatment group subjects were conducted by appointment at the subject's home or at a senior center. Interviews of treatment group subjects were conducted at the treatment centers following detoxifica-

Table 1
Demographic Characteristics of the Cross-Validation Sample

Characteristic	Treatment group[a]		Nontreatment group[b]	
Gender				
Male	168	(89%)	123	(54%)
Female	20	(11%)	104	(46%)
Race				
White	166	(88%)	211	(93%)
Black	10	(5%)	12	(5%)
Hispanic	2	(1%)	0	
Native American	10	(5%)	3	(1%)
Employment status				
Full-time	32	(17%)	16	(7%)
Part-time	13	(7%)	20	(9%)
Retired or unemployed	144	(76%)	187	(84%)
Mean age, yr	59.6		69.9	
Mean education, yr	11.7		13.6	

[a]$n = 189$.
[b]$n = 227$.
Note. Frequencies may total less than sample size due to missing responses from 1–4 subjects. Percentages may not total 100% because of rounding.

tion, if any, and when the treatment program staff had determined the individual was ready. For those unable to read, the questions were read to them. This was necessary for less than 2% of all subjects. Subjects were free to decline to respond to individual questions.

Results

Three forms of the PDSS were developed and validated. The PDSS–F(ull) is a 34-item instrument which assesses both the number and extent of problems experienced by the respondent. The PDSS–D(ichotomous) is the same instrument, scored only for number of problems. The PDSS–S(hort) is a 10-item scale. In the cross-validation sample, the reliability of both versions of the long questionnaire exceeded .98; the reliability of the PDSS–S was .95.

Questionnaire items are listed by domain in Table 2. The response scale for each item was "Never," "Occasionally," "Fairly Often," and "Very Often;" in all cases, the time period referred to was "In the Past 12 Months."

The cross-validation data were used to assess the utility of the scales in identifying problem drinkers (individuals in alcohol treatment programs)

Table 2
Scale Items by Domain

Domain	Item number	Item[a]
Consumption		
Context/timing	4.	How often have you drank alcoholic beverages when alone?
Amount	28.	How often have you become intoxicated?
Treatment	32.	How often have you gone to someone for help about your drinking?
	34.	How often have you attended an AA (Alcoholics Anonymous) meeting?
Dependence symptoms		
Use	5.	How often have you tried to hide your drinking?
	22.	How often have you kept drinking after promising yourself that you would stop?
Availability	12.	How often have you been uncomfortable because alcohol was not available?
Physical symptoms	11.	How often have you found that you can drink more without feeling the effects as much?
	31.	How often have you had tremors or shakes related to drinking?
Priorities	24.	How often have you gone without things you needed or wanted in order to drink?
Negative consequences		
Social relationships	6.	How often have you felt alone and isolated because of your drinking?
	10.	How often have you had problems with friends or family members because of your drinking?
	13.	How often have you felt others thought less highly of you because of your drinking?
	17.	How often have you had a friend or family member worry or complain about your drinking?
	20.	How often have you made excuses to someone about your drinking?
	33.	How often have you felt that the people who know you best think you have a drinking problem?

Table 2 *(continued)*

Domain	Item number	Item[a]
Health concerns	1.	How often have you had a doctor or other health worker express concern about your drinking?
Neglected responsibilities	9.	How often have you failed to take care of personal or household chores because of drinking?
Missed events/activities	14.	How often have you avoided an activity or event because of your drinking?
Personal thoughts	7.	<u>How often have you felt you ought to cut down on your drinking?</u>
	8.	<u>How often have you regretted your drinking?</u>
	18.	How often have you felt you were drinking too much for your own good?
	21.	How often have you felt you'd have fewer problems if you drank less?
	25.	How often have you thought you were losing control of your drinking?
Lapses	26.	How often have you lost or misplaced something because of drinking?
Mental state/mood	2.	How often have you felt drowsy after drinking?
	15.	How often have you had trouble remembering things because of your drinking?
	23.	How often have you felt worried after drinking?
Self-esteem	16.	<u>How often have you had bad thoughts about yourself because of your drinking?</u>
	19.	How often have you felt bad or guilty about your drinking?
Benefits		
Tension reduction	27.	How often have you drank alcoholic beverages when you got angry?
Pain reduction	3.	How often have you felt that drinking would soothe your aches and pains?
Escape	29.	<u>How often have you drank alcoholic beverages when you had nothing else to do?</u>
	30.	How often have you drank when you felt lonely?

[a]Underlined items constitute the PDSS–S.

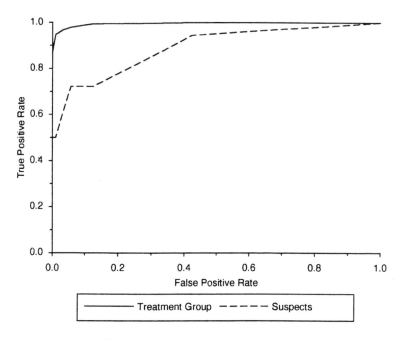

Fig. 1. ROC curves for the PDSS–S.

and nontreatment program respondents suspected of having a drinking problem. Suspects were persons whose self-reported consumption in the past month included six or more drinks on any single occasion; 18 respondents were so classified.

Using a score of 3 and above on the PDSS–S as the criterion for problem drinking, this instrument correctly classified 97.9% of the treatment group respondents (scale sensitivity) and 94.3% of the no problem respondents (scale specificity). This cutoff score classified 72.2% of the suspects as problem drinkers. A criterion score of 9 and above on both versions of the longer questionnaire (PDSS–D and PDSS–F) had equal or slightly better classification values.

A statistic for summarizing the diagnostic utility of an instrument is the area under the receiver operating characteristic (ROC) curve.[88,89] The area bounded by the ROC curve represents the probability that two randomly chosen respondents, one each from the "diseased" group and the control group, are correctly classified by the diagnostic instrument. Two such curves for the PDSS–S are displayed in Fig. 1. The ability of this instrument to contrast treatment group respondents from no problem group respondents is .996; its ability to distinguish suspects from no problem group respondents is an impressive .892.

Convergent validity of this instrument is evident in that the PDSS–S is related to other measures of problem drinking ($r = .86$ with the MAST; $r = .91$ with the CAGE). Two approaches were taken to examining the instrument's potential superiority to these measures. Areas under the ROC curves for distinguishing treatment group respondents for the PDSS-S, the PDSS-D, the MAST, and the CAGE, were .996, .998, .983, and .980, respectively. Thus, all four measures did an excellent job in this sample. The PDSS measures demonstrated some superiority with respect to identifying suspects. These ROC values were .892, .915, .828, and .855, respectively.

The ability of the PDSS to correctly classify respondents into the two known groups of alcohol treatment subjects and nontreatment subjects was further examined by conducting discriminant analyses. This approach permitted controlling for demographic characteristics that differed between these two groups. Treatment group respondents were both younger and more likely to be male than nontreatment group respondents. Controlling for age and gender, the misclassification rates of the PDSS–S, the PDSS–D, the MAST, and the CAGE were .051, .041, .068, and .091, respectively. The error rate reported for the PDSS–S includes 11 nontreatment subjects misclassified as problem drinkers; of these, 9 were suspects. The PDSS–S thus appears to be a very promising screening tool.

Use of the PDSS

Persons scoring 3 or higher on the PDSS–S or 9 or above on the longer questionnaire (PDSS–D and PDSS–F) have responded in a manner similar to persons in alcohol treatment programs, and referral for treatment is very likely appropriate. But any positive score on the PDSS is suggestive of some problem and warrants further consideration and possible intervention. For screening purposes, the shorter form PDSS–S has demonstrated nearly the same effectiveness as the longer forms. Dichotomous scoring is recommended for screening. A criterion score on the PDSS identifies problem drinkers, however, a low score should not be interpreted as indicating that an individual's drinking practices are necessarily safe.

Conclusions and Recommendations

1. Although we believe that there are special issues and difficulties related to the identification of older problem drinkers, we contend that these have more to do with mistaken beliefs, age prejudice, and inadequate practices than to the inherent characteristics of older people, their circumstances, or a lack of useful screening instruments. The unique problems associated with screening the elderly are largely manageable, and are only minor in relation to the seriousness of problems resulting from a failure to identify and intervene.

2. Evidence regarding the MAST and CAGE is encouraging for their use with older persons, even though neither was developed specifically for the elderly. Still, it seems clear that the MAST and CAGE are not interchangeable,[46] and neither is without limitations. Among these limitations are shared emphasis on active alcoholism at any time in the person's life, as opposed to more current and more broadly conceptualized hazardous or problematic drinking.
3. Screening questionnaires for identifying problem drinking have been developed with, and specifically for, older persons and use items designed to address expressed concerns regarding age. The limited evidence available suggests these age-specific screens perform very well with older persons, and somewhat better than do the nonage-specific instruments.
4. The response format of the PDSS, which permits the respondent to minimize without denying an alcohol problem, may help to reduce the impact on screening of any tendency toward denial. This possibility, however, has not been directly tested. With all such instruments, including the PDSS, the use of collaterals or other supporting evidence is recommended, when practical.
5. In attempting to identify those older persons whose alcohol use places them at special risk, the target focus needs to be broader than identifying alcoholics. The criteria for what is risky should generally be lowered for the elderly,[15,20] but also be individualized in relation to such variables as health and medication status. It is possible to identify individuals as probable high-risk drinkers with a questionnaire such as the PDSS, but more information is required to determine what might be dangerous drinking, given a person's individual circumstances. Comprehensive assessment is best with older persons, assessment that includes a screen such as the PDSS, a determination of alcohol intake and patterns of use, and a consideration of health factors, including prescription and over-the-counter medications.

Acknowledgment

Development of the PDSS was supported by National Institute on Alcohol Abuse and Alcoholism Grant 1 R01 AA 07683.

References

[1]E. A. Chrischilles, D. J. Foley, R. B. Wallace, J. H. Lemke, T. P. Semla, J. T. Hanlon, et al. (1992) Use of medications by persons 65 and over: data from the established populations for epidemiologic studies of the elderly. *J. Gerontol. Med. Sci.* **47(5),** M137–M144.
[2]A. L. Sheahan, J. Hendricks, and J. S. Coons (1989) Drug misuse among the elderly: a covert problem. *Health Values* **13(3),** 22–29.
[3]A. Graham, T. Parren, and J. Carlos (1992) Physician failure to record alcohol use history when prescribing benzodiazepines. *J. Subst. Abuse* **4(2),** 179–185.

[4]T. F. Babor, H. R. Kranzler, and R. Kadden (1986) Issues in the definition and diagnosis of alcoholism: implications for a reformulation. *Prog. Neuro-Psychopharmacol. Biol. Psychiatry* **10**, 113–128.

[5]T. F. Babor, H. R. Kranzler, and R. Lauermann (1989) Early detection of harmful alcohol consumption: comparison of clinical laboratory and self-report screening procedures. *Addict. Behav.* **14**, 139–157.

[6]G. R. Jacobson (1989) A comprehensive approach to pretreatment evaluation: I. Detection, assessment and diagnosis of alcoholism, in *Handbook of Alcoholism Treatment Approaches*. R. K. Hester and W. R. Miller, eds. Pergamon, Elmsford, NY, pp. 17–53.

[7]R. E. Tarter, H. B. Moss, A. Arria, A. Mezzich, and M. M. Vanyukov (1992) The psychiatric diagnosis of alcoholism: critique and proposed reformulation. *Alcohol. Clin. Exper. Res.* **16**, 106–116.

[8]R. Watson (1989) *Diagnosis of Alcohol Abuse*. CRC, Boca Raton, FL.

[9]J. H. Mendelson and N. K. Mello (1985) *The Diagnosis and Treatment of Alcoholism*. McGraw-Hill, New York.

[10]R. Caetano (1987) When will we have a standard concept of alcohol dependence? *Br. J. Addict.* **82**, 601–607.

[11]R. M. Atkinson (1988) Alcoholism in the elderly population. *Mayo Clin. Proc.* **63**, 825–828.

[12]R. M. Atkinson (1990) Aging and alcohol use disorder diagnostic issues in the elderly. *Int. Psychogeriatr.* **2(1)**, 55–72.

[13]K. Graham (1986) Identifying and measuring alcohol abuse among the elderly: serious problems with existing instrumentation. *J. Stud. Alcohol* **47**, 322–326.

[14]A. W. Lawson (1988) Substance abuse problems of the elderly: considerations for treatment and prevention, in *Alcoholism and Substance Abuse in Special Populations*. G. W. Lawson and A. W. Lawson, eds. Aspen, Gaithersburg, MD, pp. 95–113.

[15]M. Schuckit (1990) Introduction: assessment and treatment strategies with the late life alcoholic. *J. Geriatr. Psychiatry* **23(3)**, 83–89.

[16]E. W. Pruzinsky (1987) Alcohol and the elderly: an overview of problems in the elderly and implications for social work practice. *J. Gerontol. Soc. Work* **11**, 81–93.

[17]S. Widner and A. Zeichner (1991) Alcohol abuse in the elderly: review of epidemiology research and treatment. *Clin. Gerontol.* **11(1)**, 3–20.

[18]R. C. Abrams and G. Alexopoulos (1991) Geriatric addictions, in *Clinical Textbook of Addictive Disorders*. R. Frances and S. Miller, eds. Guilford, New York, pp. 347–365.

[19]G. Caracci and N. Miller (1991) Epidemiology and diagnosis of alcoholism in the elderly (a review). *Int. J. Geriatr. Psychiatry* **6**, 511–515.

[20]D. Bienenfeld (1987) Alcoholism in the elderly. *Am. Fam. Phys.* **36**, 163–169.

[21]K. Hesse and J. Savitsky (1987) The elderly, in *Alcoholism: A Guide for the Primary Care Physician*. H. Barnes, M. Aronson, and T. Delbanco, eds. Springer-Verlag, New York, pp. 167–175.

[22]D. G. Blazer and M. R. Pennybacker (1984) Epidemiology of alcoholism in the elderly, in *Alcoholism in the Elderly: Social and Biomedical Issues*. J. T. Hartford and T. Samorajski, eds. Raven, New York, pp. 25–33.

[23]H. W. Gruchow, J. Barboriak, and K. Sobocinski (1989) Alcohol consumption and abuse among women and the elderly, in *Diagnosis of Alcohol Abuse*. R. R. Watson, ed. CRC, Boca Raton, FL, pp. 217–230.

[24]R. J. Curtis, G. Geller, E. Stokes, D. Levine, and R. Moore (1989) Characteristics diagnosis and treatment of alcoholism in elderly patients. *J. Am. Geriatr. Soc.* **37,** 310–316.

[25]B. Carruth (1973) Toward a definition of problem drinking among older people: conceptual and methodological considerations, in *Alcoholism and Problem Drinking Among Older Persons.* E. Williams and B. Carruth, eds. National Technical Information Services, Springfield, VA, pp. 110–114.

[26]J. W. Finney and R. H. Moos (1984) Life stressors and problem drinking among older adults, in *Recent Developments in Alcoholism,* vol. 2. M. Galanter, ed. Plenum, New York, pp. 267–288.

[27]American Psychiatric Association (1987) *Diagnostic and Statistical Manual of Mental Disorders* (3rd ed., rev.). Author, Washington, DC.

[28]H. A. Mulford and J. L. Fitzgerald (1992) Elderly vs. young problem drinkers, do they indicate a need for special programs for the elderly. *J. Stud. Alcohol* **53,** 601–610.

[29]M. Willenbring and W. D. Spring (1988) Evaluating alcohol use in elders. *Generations* **12(4),** 27–31.

[30]R. M. Atkinson, L. Ganzini, and M. Bernstein (1992) Alcohol and substance-use disorders in the elderly, in *Handbook of Mental Health and Aging,* 2nd ed. J. E. Birren, ed. Academic, Boston, pp. 515–555.

[31]R. H. Moos, J. R. Mertens, and P. L. Brennan (1992) Patterns of diagnosis and treatment among late-middle-aged and older substance abuse patients. *J. Stud. Alcohol* **54,** 479–487.

[32]M. D. Hayward and M. C. Liu (1992) Men and women in their retirement years: a demographic profile, in *Families and Retirement.* M. Szinovacz, D. J. Ekerdt, and B. H. Vinick, eds. Sage, London, pp. 25–50.

[33]D. F. Hultsch and R. A. Dixon (1990) Learning and memory in aging, in *Handbook of the Psychology of Aging,* 3rd ed. J. E. Birren and K. W. Schaie, eds. Academic, New York, pp. 258–274.

[34]J. A. Sugar and J. M. McDowd (1992) Memory, learning and attention, in *Handbook of Mental Health and Aging,* 2nd ed. J. E. Birren, R. B. Sloane, and G. D. Cohen, eds. Academic, New York, pp. 307–337.

[35]L. W. Poon (1989) What do we know about the aging of cognitive abilities in everyday life?, in *Everyday Cognition in Adulthood and Late Life.* L. W. Poon, D. C. Rubin, and B. A. Wilson, eds. Cambridge University Press, New York, pp. 129–132.

[36]J. C. Anthony and A. Aboraya (1992) The epidemiology of selected mental disorders in later life, in *Handbook of Mental Health and Aging,* 2nd ed. J. E. Birren, R. B. Sloane, and G. D. Cohen, eds. Academic, New York, pp. 28–73.

[37]M. J. Gilewski and E. M. Zelinski (1986) Questionnaire assessment of memory complaints, in *Handbook for Clinical Memory Assessment of Older Adults.* L. W. Poon, ed. American Psychological Association, Washington, DC, pp. 93–107.

[38]R. Bilder and J. Kane (1989) Assessment of organic mental disorders, in *Measuring Mental Illness: Psychometric Assessment for Clinicians.* S. Wetzer, ed. American Psychiatric Press, Washington, DC, pp. 183–208.

[39]M. F. Folstein, S. E. Folstein, and P. R. McHugh (1975) Mini-mental state: a practical method for grading the cognitive state of patients for the clinician. *J. Psychiatr. Res.* **12,** 189–198.

[40]E. Pfeiffer (1974) Short portable mental status questionnaire for the measurement of organic brain deficits in elderly patients. *J. Am. Geriatr. Soc.* **23,** 433–441.

[41]T. P. Beresford, F. C. Blow, K. J. Brower, and K. Singer (1988) Clinical applications screening for alcoholism. *Prev. Med.* **17**, 653–663.

[42]T. Babor, R. Stephens, and A. Marlatt (1987) Verbal reports methods in clinical research on alcoholism: response bias and its minimization. *J. Stud. Alcohol* **48**, 410–424.

[43]L. Midanik (1982) Over reports of recent alcohol consumption in a clinical population: a validity study. *Drug Alcohol Depend.* **9**, 101–110.

[44]T. O'Farrell and S. Maitso (1987) The utility of self report and biological measures of alcohol consumption in alcoholism treatment outcome studies. *Adv. Behav. Res. Ther.* **9**, 91–125.

[45]L. Davis and R. Morse (1987) Patient-spouse agreement on the drinking behaviors of alcoholics. *Mayo Clin. Proc.* **62**, 689–694.

[46]D. J. Lee and R. S. DeFrank (1988) Interrelationships among self-reported alcohol intake, physiological indices and alcoholism screening measures. *J. Stud. Alcohol* **49**, 532–537.

[47]P. Lemmens, E. S. Tan, and R. L. Knibble (1992) Measuring quantity and frequency of drinking in a general population survey: a comparison of five indices. *J. Stud. Alcohol* **53**, 476–486.

[48]L. Midanik (1992) Reliability of self-reported alcohol consumption before and after December. *Addict. Behav.* **17**, 179–184.

[49]P .F. Smith, P. L. Remington, and D. Williamson (1990) A comparison of alcohol sales data with survey data on self-reported alcohol use in 21 states. *Am. J. Pub. Health* **80**, 309–312.

[50]L. Sobell, M. Sobell, D. Riley, and R. Schuller (1988) The reliability of alcohol abusers' self-reports of drinking and life events that occurred in the distant past. *J. Stud. Alcohol* **49**, 225–232.

[51]J. A. Gladsjo, J. A. Tucker, J. Hawkins, and R. Y. Vuchinich (1992) Adequacy of recall of drinking patterns and event occurrences associated with natural recovery from alcohol problems. *Addict. Behav.* **17**, 347–358.

[52]J. A. Tucker and R. E. Virchinich (1991) Agreement between subject and collateral verbal reports of alcohol consumption in older adults. *J. Stud. Alcohol* **52**, 148–155.

[53]E. A. O'Keefe, N. J. Talley, E. G. Tangalos, and A. R. Zinsmeister (1992) A bowel symptom questionnaire for the elderly. *J. Gerontol. Med. Sci.* **47**, M116–M121.

[54]D. B. Reuben, L. Laliberte, and J. Hiris (1990) A hierarchical exercise scale to measure function at the advanced activities of daily living (AADL) level. *J. Am. Geriatr. Soc.* **38**, 855–861.

[55]D. B. Reuben, A. L. Siu, and S. Kimpau (1992) The predictive validity of self-report and performance-based measures of function and health. *J. Gerontol. Med. Sci.* **47**, M106–M110.

[56]C. D. Sherbourne and L. S. Merideth (1992) Quality of self-report data: a comparison of older and younger chronically ill patients. *J. Gerontol. Soc. Sci.* **47**, S204–S211.

[57]W. D. Spector, S. Katz, and J. B. Murphy (1987) The hierarchical relationship between activities of daily living and instrumental activities of daily living. *J. Chron. Disabil.* **40**, 481–490.

[58]A. B. Ford, S. J. Folmar, R. B. Salmon, J. H. Medalie, A. W. Roy, and S. S. Galazka (1988) Health and function in the very old. *J. Am. Geriatr. Soc.* **36**, 187–197.

[59]D. Mayfield, G. McLeod, and P. Hall (1974) The CAGE questionnaire: validation of a new alcoholism screening instrument. *Am. J. Psychiatry* **131**, 1121–1123.

[60]M. L. Selzer (1971) The Michigan Alcoholism Screening Test: the quest for a new diagnostic instrument. *Am. J. Psychiatry* **127**, 89–94.

[61]F. C. Blow, K. J. Brower, J. E. Schulenberg, L. M. Demo-Dananberg, J. P. Young, and T. P. Beresford (1992) The Michigan Alcoholism Screening Test–Geriatric Version (MAST–G): a new elderly-specific screening instrument. *Alcohol. Clin. Exper. Res.* **16**, 372.

[62]J. Ewing (1984) Detecting alcoholism: the CAGE questionnaire. *JAMA* **252**, 1905–1907.

[63]T. Beresford, F. Blow, E. Hill, K. Singer, and M. Lucey (1990) Comparison of CAGE questionnaire and computer-assisted laboratory profiles in screening for covert alcoholism. *Lancet* **336**, 482–485.

[64]D. G. Buchsbaum, R. G. Buchanan, R. M. Centor, S. H. Schnoll, and M. J. Lawton (1991) Screening for alcohol abuse using CAGE scores and likelihood ratios. *Ann. Intern. Med.* **115**, 774–777.

[65]B. Bush, S. Shaw, P. Cleary, T. Delbanco, and M. Aronson (1987) Screening for alcohol abuse using the CAGE questionnaire. *Am. J. Med.* **82**, 231–235.

[66]M. King (1986) At-risk drinking among general practice attenders: validation of the CAGE questionnaire. *Psychol. Med.* **16**, 213–217.

[67]R. Gonzalez-Menedez, I. Donaire-Calabuch, E. Uliver-Valesquez, and J. Farran-Leyva (1989) CAGE and MAST abbreviated questionnaire in an internal medicine service: sensitivity and specificity according to direct or family information sources. *Revista-del-Hospital-Psiquiartrico-de-La-Habana* **30**, 197–207.

[68]L. W. Glaze and P. G. Coggan (1987) Efficacy of an alcoholism self-report questionnaire in a residency clinic. *J. Fam. Prac.* **25**, 60–64.

[69]B. L. Niles and B. S. McGrady (1991) Detection of alcohol problems in a hospital setting. *Addict. Behav.* **16**, 223–233.

[70]H. D. Mischke and R. Venneri (1987) Reliability and validity of the MAST, Mortimer-Filkins questionnaire and CAGE in DWI assessment. *J. Stud. Alcohol* **48**, 492–501.

[71]E. J. Waterson and I. M. Murray-Lyon (1988) Are the CAGE questions outdated? *Br. J. Addict.* **83**, 1113–1118.

[72]D. G. Buchsbaum, R. G. Buchanan, J. Welsh, R. M. Centor, and S. H. Schnoll (1992) Screening for drinking disorders in the elderly using the CAGE questionnaire. *J. Am. Geriatr. Soc.* **40**, 661–665.

[73]L. N. Robins, J. E. Helzer, J. Croughan, and J. S. Ratcliff (1981) National Institute of Mental Health Diagnostic Interview Schedule: its history, characteristics, and validity. *Arch. Gen. Psychiatry* **38**, 381–389.

[74]American Psychiatric Association (1980) *Diagnostic and Statistical Manual of Mental Disorders* (3rd ed.). Author, Washington, DC.

[75]A. D. Pokorny, B. A. Miller, and H. B. Kaplin (1972) The brief MAST: a shortened version of the Michigan Alcoholism Screening Test. *Am. J. Psychiatry* **129**, 342–345.

[76]M. L. Selzer, A. Vinokur, and L. A. Van Rooijen (1975) Self-administered Short Michigan Alcoholism Screening Test. *J. Stud. Alcohol* **36**, 117–126.

[77]G. R. Jacobson (1989) Identification of problem drinkers and alcoholics, in *Diagnosis of Alcohol Abuse*. R. R. Watson, ed. CRC, Boca Raton, FL, pp. 177–200.

[78]R. M. Morse and R. D. Hurt (1979) Screening for alcoholism. *JAMA* **242**, 2688–2690.

[79]R. D. Hurt, R. M. Morse, and W. M. Swenson (1980) Diagnosis of alcoholism with a self-administered alcoholism screening test: results with 1,002 consecutive patients receiving general examinations. *Mayo Clin. Proc.* **55,** 365–370.

[80]G. R. Jacobson (1983) Detection, assessment, and diagnosis of alcoholism: current techniques, in *Recent Developments in Alcoholism,* vol 1. M. Galanter, ed. Plenum, New York, pp. 377–413.

[81]D. J. Lettieri, J. E. Nelson, and M. A. Sayers (1985) *Treatment Handbook Series: 2. Alcoholism Treatment Assessment Research Instruments.* National Institute on Alcohol Abuse and Alcoholism, Rockville, MD.

[82]L. Morey and P. Martin (1989) Assessment of alcoholism and substance abuse, in *Measuring Mental Illness: Psychometric Assessment for Clinicians.* S. Wetzler, ed. American Psychiatric Press, Washington, DC, pp. 161–181.

[83]M. L. Willenbring, K. J. Christensen, W. D. Spring, and R. Rasmussen (1987) Alcoholism screening in the elderly. *J. Am. Geriatr. Soc.* **35,** 864–869.

[84]B. Yersin, Y. Tusconi, F. Gutzwiller, and P. Magnessat (1989) Accuracy of the Michigan Alcoholism Screening Test for screening of alcoholism in patients of a medical department. *Arch. Int. Med.* **149,** 2071–2074.

[85]E. Tabisz, M. Badger, R. Meatherall, W. Jacyk, D. Fuchs, and R. Grymonpre (1991) Identification of chemical abuse in the elderly admitted to emergency. *Clin. Gerontol.* **11,** 27–38.

[86]P. D. Cleary, M. Miller, B. T. Bush, M. M. Warburg, T. L. Delbanco, and M. D. Aronson (1988) Prevalence and recognition of alcohol abuse in a primary care population. *Am. J. Med.* **85,** 466–470.

[87]H. E. Ross, D. R. Gavin, and H. A. Skinner (1990) Diagnostic validity of the MAST and the alcohol dependence scale in the assessment of DSM–III alcohol disorders. *J. Stud. Alcohol* **51,** 506–513.

[88]J. A. Hanley and B. J. McNeil (1982) The meaning and use of the area under a receiver operating characteristic (ROC) curve. *Radiology* **143,** 29–36.

[89]J. K. Hsiao, J. J. Bartko, and W. Z. Potter (1989) Diagnosing diagnoses: receiver operating characteristic methods and psychiatry. *Arch. Gen. Psychiatry* **46,** 664–667.

Youth, Alcohol, and Automobiles

Attitudes and Behaviors

Mary-Ellen Fortini

Introduction

It is well established that young drivers are at high risk for accident involvement[1] and for alcohol-related fatal crashes.[2,3] In fact, alcohol-related motor vehicle crashes are the number one cause of death for American youth.[4]

Motor vehicle crashes accounted for over 40% of all teenage deaths in 1986; more than half of these were alcohol related. According to 1985 Fatal Accident Reporting System (FARS) data, 16–24 yr olds have the highest rates of alcohol-related fatal crashes per mile traveled.[2]

Furthermore, of fatal accidents involving young drivers, 36% occurred in accidents in which at least one driver had been drinking.[5] Of particular concern is the fact that a greater percentage of young drivers, as compared to older drivers, are involved in fatal crashes at lower blood alcohol concentrations (BACs).[5,6]

From 1982–1987, there was a reduction in the proportion of drivers involved in fatal crashes who were intoxicated (decrease for all drivers 17%), especially for 16–19-yr-old drivers (34% decrease). Although this is encouraging and interesting, the fact remains that fatal accident involvement per miles driven is significantly higher for teenagers than all other age groups. For drivers age 25–34, there was little or no reduction. Fell and Nash[7] suggested that the reductions are a result of increased efforts in education and awareness, tougher laws and stricter enforcement, higher minimum legal

From: *Drug and Alcohol Abuse Reviews, Vol. 7: Alcohol, Cocaine, and Accidents*
Ed.: R. R. Watson ©1995 Humana Press Inc., Totowa, NJ

drinking age, interventions, a decline in the population of youthful drivers, and a decrease in per capita alcohol consumption.

A number of reasons for the elevated risk of teenagers have been proposed, the most common being adolescents' inexperience with both drinking and driving, making the combination especially dangerous.[6,8] Other possibilities include high risk-taking behavior, immaturity, and poor judgment.[6]

Methodological Limitations

Before discussing adolescent drinking and driving it is important to discuss a number of limitations of the studies presented. First, one of the difficulties in comparing studies on youth involvement in alcohol-related injuries and deaths is the inconsistency of age categories. Categories defined as young drivers have included all drivers under 30 and drivers ages 16–19, 16–24, and 18–25, making comparisons across studies difficult.

A second limitation has been the definition of the term driving while impaired. Most studies on drinking and driving among youth rely on self-report, using various terms in the surveys: impaired driving, driving when you thought you were over the legal alcohol limit, and drunken driving. There has been no systematic examination done on the differences between these terms.

Perhaps the most commonly cited problem with studies is that, with the exception of fatal accident data, there has been a reliance on self-report. It has been generally accepted among researchers that individuals over-report positive behaviors and under-report negative behaviors. Survey data are commonly criticized on these grounds. Although there is probably limited value of self-report in providing accurate estimates of the frequency of particular driving behaviors for individuals, self-reported behavior is significantly related to observed behavior and is therefore valid.[9]

Alcohol Consumption
Among Adolescents

In a national health survey of students,[10] over 87% of 10th graders reported using alcohol in their lifetime, with 13% reporting frequent use in the past 30 d. In Fortini,[11] 76% of high school students reported drinking alcohol at least once in the previous year. Of those students who drank alcohol in the previous year, 19% reported that they generally drink five or more drinks per sitting, and 25% reported that they drink their usual amount at least once a week. Students were also asked to report the quantity and frequency of alcohol consumption on those occasions in which they drank more than their usual amount. Of those who drank in the previous year, 53% said they drank five or more drinks per sitting, with 6% reporting they drank more than their usual amount at least once per week. Thirty-two percent reported drinking more than their usual amount at least once a month.

In household surveys of 13–18 yr olds, Zucker and Harford[12] found that 60% of adolescents were drinkers, with 6% classified as heavier drinkers. Heavier drinkers were defined as those who drink at least once a week and typically drink five or more drinks per sitting. Not surprisingly, more males than females were drinkers and heavier drinkers. Fifty-nine percent of 18-yr-old boys classified as moderate-heavier or heavier drinkers. Twenty-two percent of the sample reported drunkenness at least once a month (26% of the boys and 17% of the girls). Windle[10] also reported that 36.6% of the 10th-grade population in the national survey reported consuming five or more drinks on at least one occasion in the 2 wk previous to the survey.

In a Canadian study on drinking and driving,[13] the younger age group (ages 16–19) was more likely than the older (ages 20–24) to report drinking within the previous year, although the older Canadians reported drinking more frequently. Three percent of the younger and about 8% of the older Canadians reported drinking four or more times per week. The quantity data looked considerably different, however, with the number of drinks consumed in the previous week the highest for those ages 20–24 and decreasing steadily for older groups. Males drank over twice as much as females in the younger groups.

There was also a difference in age distribution among drinking and nondrinking drivers, with over 60% of all drinking drivers between the ages of 16 and 34. When comparing drinking with nondrinking drivers on average weekly alcohol consumption, drinking drivers always reported a higher rate than nondrinking drivers. However, the difference between drinking and nondrinking drivers was much greater for young drivers. The consumption for nondrinking drivers remains relatively constant across all age groups (except ages 55–64). However, the average weekly consumption is much higher for the younger drinking drivers than for older drinking drivers.

High-Risk Driving Behaviors

Young males report engaging in all high-risk driving behaviors more than females,[14] and young drivers take more driving risks than do older drivers.[9] A number of driving behaviors have been identified as high risk and, in general, 16–24-yr-old drivers engage in these behaviors more frequently than older age groups. These behaviors include: driving through

yellow lights, passing at an intersection, following too closely, and changing lanes abruptly.[9]

Safety Belt Use

It is well known that those wearing safety belts are less likely to be
injured in the event of a crash. In a report of 1991 fatality facts, the National
Center for Statistics and Analysis reported that among occupants of vehicles
involved in fatal crashes, safety belt use was lowest among those between
10 and 24 yr of age. However, Jonah and Dawson[9] found that young drivers
reported using safety belts more often than those ages 21–24.

Nighttime Driving

The majority of alcohol-related incidents occur in the evening.
Although young drivers do only 20% of their driving at night, over 50% of
their accident fatalities occur in the nighttime.[15] In the San Diego County
student survey,[11] students were asked how frequently they drove after
10 PM in the past month. Fewer than 50% reported they drove at least one
weeknight (Sunday through Thursday) in the previous month, whereas over
75% reported driving at least one weekend night (Friday or Saturday).

Driving While Impaired

Nearly 42% of the 18–24-yr-old population in a national survey in
1983 reported driving one or more times while impaired by alcohol.[14]
Although 16–24 yr olds account for less than 30% of all drinking drivers in
Canada, 60% of those surveyed in this age group reported that they drink
and drive.[12]

Analysis by Fortini[11] showed that, of students who reported drinking
alcohol, 23% reported driving when they thought at the time they were
probably over the legal limit at least once; 4% reported doing so 10 or more
times. With regard to other high-risk behaviors, 29% reported driving after
drinking more than their usual amount of alcohol, 34% reported driving
within 1 h of their last drink sometimes or more often, and 80% believed
they could drink three or more drinks within 1 h and still drive safely.

Even though adolescents are driving impaired at high rates, the rate of
juvenile driving under the influence (DUI) arrests and convictions are very
low.[16] Young drivers are arrested for driving while intoxicated (DWI) at
significantly lower rates than their incidence in alcohol-related crashes.[17]

Vegega and Klitzner[18] examined situational risk factors associated with
DWI and with riding with an impaired driver. Not surprisingly, drinking
was the key situational variable in driving while impaired. Those surveyed
reported that they drove because they were the most sober in the group. The
second most reported situational variable was the need to get somewhere or

get someone else somewhere (usually home). This was more true for females than for males. Fortini[11] reported similar findings. More females than males reported promising someone a ride home was likely to influence their decision to drive after drinking.

Riding with an Impaired Driver

In addition to taking many risks as driver, 40% of the students in the San Diego County study reported that they have been a passenger in a car in which the driver was intoxicated.[11] For factors associated with riding with an impaired driver, Vegega and Klitzner[18] found a key variable was the need to get somewhere (home).

Other Behaviors

Young drivers (15–19) arrested for DUI in Massachusetts in February 1979 were found to have a higher than predicted frequency of other charges, such as, operating to endanger, unauthorized use of a motor vehicle, property damage, personal injury, speeding, reckless driving, and public violations.[19]

Accident Involvement

Alcohol use by youth has been singled out as a major cause of head trauma and subsequent impairment or death in Canada.[20] Young males are at a much greater risk than females for crashes[1] and for alcohol-related crashes and fatalities.[2,21] Stoddard and Rothe[5] reported that 16–19-yr-old males have the highest crash rate per miles driven and that drivers under age 25 are over-represented in alcohol-related accidents.

The increased risk is also apparent at lower BACs. Zador[22] reported that, using males 25 yr and older as the criterion group, males ages 16–20 had an increased fatal injury risk of 12.3 at BACs between 0.05 and 0.09%. Even though young males are generally seen as having the greatest risk, Zador also found that females ages 16–20 in the 0.05–0.09% BAC range had an increased risk of 21.3 relative to males 25 and over.

Because adolescents are relatively inexperienced drivers, they are a high-risk group for accident involvement. In San Diego County,[11] 31% reported they had one or more accidents as the driver during their lifetime (11% had two or more). Of those reporting accidents, 4% said the accident occurred within 1 h or so of drinking alcohol.

Similar results are found in Canada, with the highest percentage of drivers involved in crashes in the 20–24 age group.[13] The percentage of both the death rate and injury rate from motor vehicle accidents was highest among 15–24 yr olds in both 1978 and 1985.[23]

On a per capita basis, 18-yr-old male and 19-yr-female drivers account for the largest number of car-driver fatalities within each gender.[21] As found in other studies, male involvement in accidents at all ages exceeds that of females.

Jonah and Dawson[9] found that drivers ages 16–20 had a much higher accident rate per kilometers driven than all other age groups. Similarly, the younger drivers had significantly more accidents in the previous 3 yr and a higher violation rate per miles driven. This group also reported a greater mean number of trips while impaired, but the authors question the validity of this finding since a number of young drivers indicated they had been driving while impaired 30 times in the previous 30 d.

Although there are a number of studies that show that young males are more involved in DUI arrests and accidents than young females, young females are a group that should be targeted for prevention efforts. In a study of changes in arrest rates and alcohol-related crashes in North Carolina,[24] Popkin reported that, from 1979–1984 for males of all age groups under 34, there was a decrease in DWIs, alcohol-related accidents, and single vehicle nighttime accidents. For females, however, the picture was dramatically different. Regarding DWI arrests rates, for 21–24 yr olds, there was an increase of 26%. Alcohol-related crashes increased 74% for 18–20 yr olds, 93% for 21–24 yr olds, and 45% for 25–34 yr olds. There were also increases in single vehicle nighttime crashes for females: 29% for 18 and under, 33% for 18–20, 43% for 21–24, and 17% for 25–34.

Actions for Reducing Crashes

A number of policy changes have been made and recommended in an effort to reduce adolescent crashes. Although some have been studied extensively, others have not.

Raising the Drinking Age

In 1985, a federal regulation was passed that required states to raise the minimum drinking age to 21 in order to receive federal highway funds. In the decade prior to that change, a number of states had already raised their minimum drinking age. The National Highway Traffic Safety Administration (NHTSA) estimates that laws increasing the minimum drinking age have saved over 12,000 lives from 1975–1991.[25] Similar findings have been reported by Blomberg,[26] Jones et al.,[27] Hingson et al.,[28] Wagenaar,[29,30] and Lillis et al.[31] This policy has not been without controversy, however. Mosher[32] questioned this policy in its attempt at discriminating against young drivers, since alcohol increases everyone's risk.

Although in general raising the drinking age has an impact on reducing young driver fatality and other alcohol-related accidents, special attention needs to be given to those areas in which bordering countries do not have similar legal drinking ages.[33,34] From 1980–1985 fatal crashes involving intoxicated teenage drivers decreased, but between 1985 and 1986 they increased 14% among 15–17 yr olds. Increasing minimum drinking age reduces fatal alcohol-related crashes among youth. *Per se* laws produce short-term effects, but only produce long-term effects if the public perceives a high likelihood that intoxicated drivers will be stopped by police. Adolescent deaths from injuries other than motor vehicle crashes also decreased when the minimum drinking age was raised.[35]

Detection Training for Officers

The NHTSA[17] suggested that driving cues for drinking and driving may be different for the younger driver and that police officers may not detect young DUIs as readily. Zylman[36] reported that there is a wide variation within states in the enforcement of traffic laws and reporting of crashes. Police agencies, prosecutors, and judges have much discretion in the interpretation and implementation of the laws that exist. This effort is one that requires further investigation and evaluation.

Other Policy Changes

The National Safety Transportation Board[37] has made a number of recommendations for policy changes. In addition to those mentioned here, they offer the following: stronger penalties for underage drinking/purchasing of alcohol, driving restrictions, and provisional youth licensing. Mosher[38] stated that policy changes must be implemented for long-term changes in drunken driving and crash rates to be effective. Among his suggestions are policy changes in: alcohol availability, price and tax policies, server intervention programs, alcohol advertising, and transportation policies. Together with individual change interventions, reductions in alcohol-related crashes by youth may be possible.

Attitudes Toward Alcohol and Drinking and Driving

Relative to older drivers, those between the ages of 16 and 24 are more likely than older drivers to believe that risky behaviors are less dangerous.[9] Further, younger drivers perceived safety countermeasures to be less effective in reducing casualties.

A Canadian study[12] found that only 4% of Canadians surveyed participated in a designated driver program and that over 70% of those who did participate were between the ages of 20 and 34. They also reported that the lowest involvement in campaigns against drinking and driving was among those between 20 and 34.

Leigh[39] suggested that alcohol expectancies are a component of attitudes toward alcohol and, as such, are predictive of drinking behaviors. Individuals who hold positive expectations about alcohol consumption are more likely to consume alcohol. A number of studies have been conducted to identify both positive and negative beliefs about alcohol effects[39,40] and outcomes of driving after drinking,[11] again finding a correlation between positive beliefs and consumption. Other studies that have examined the relationship between alcohol expectancies and drinking behaviors,[41] and risk-taking behaviors[42] have found similar results.

Theoretical Models for Examining Adolescent Drinking and Driving

Much of the work on adolescent drinking and driving has been atheoretical in nature,[43] but recent research has focused on applying psychosocial theories that incorporate attitudes to the prediction of this behavior. Two such theories have been the Problem Behavior Theory and the Theory of Reasoned Action (and the newer Theory of Planned Behavior).

Problem Behavior Theory

Research on adolescent behavior with regard to theoretical models has been dominated for the past 20 yr by the Problem Behavior Theory.[44] This model proposes three systems of influence: the Personality System, the Perceived Environment System, and the Behavior System. Within each system variables reflect factors that lead to or control engaging in problem behaviors. Combined, these factors result in problem behavior proneness or risk.[45] Proneness refers to involvement in problem behaviors other than the one being predicted.

A premise of the theory is that there is a syndrome of problem behaviors that are intercorrelated and all serve similar psychosocial functions, such as affiliation with peers, asserting independence, and establishing personal identity, among others. Problem Behavior Theory has been used by Jessor and colleagues to examine a number of behaviors, including problem drinking, marijuana use, cigaret smoking, and risky driving.[45–48]

Beirness and Simpson[49] found that crash involvement by youth could be considered part of a general syndrome of high-risk and problem behavior among adolescents. In a 4-yr longitudinal study, they found differences between adolescents who were involved in crashes and those who were not on variables in each of the three systems. Of great importance, they also found that the lifestyle factors that are predictive of crash involvement are present prior to the age of licensing.

These findings were supported by Johnson and White.[50] In a study of 556 adolescents ages 18–21, evidence supported the idea that drinking and driving is part of a syndrome of risk-taking behaviors. It was most often engaged in by youth who used alcohol frequently and as a coping strategy. The use of alcohol as a coping mechanism was the strongest predictor of driving under the influence in a regression analysis. Path analysis revealed that risk-taking orientation was the strongest predictor of DUI both directly and mediated through drinking to cope.

Theory of Reasoned Action/Planned Behavior

The Theory of Reasoned Action was first proposed to explain the relationship between attitudes and behaviors.[51,52] According to this theory, an individual's *intention* to perform a particular behavior is the most immediate predictor of that behavior. Further, there are two determinants of intention. The first is the *attitude toward performing the behavior* in question. This refers not to the individual's general attitudes but specifically to attitudes toward engaging in the behavior. The attitudinal component is determined by what the individual sees as the consequences of engaging in that behavior weighted by the evaluation of each of those consequences.

The second predictor of intention is called the *subjective norm*. This refers to the individual's perception of what people think he or she should do relative to the behavior. This component is determined by the individual's beliefs about what specific significant people think he or she should do, weighted by the individual's motivation to comply with each of those referents.

More recent work by Ajzen[53] suggested that for behaviors that are not under the volitional control of the individual, intentions can be seen less as predictors of behavior and more as "plans of action in pursuit of behavioral goals." In order to permit behavioral action, an individual must have some control over whether he or she can perform this behavior. For this reason, a third predictor of intention has been added—that of *perceived control*. The determinants of perceived control are the factors that will affect whether or not the individual will perform the behavior in question weighted by the likelihood of the occurrence of each factor. With this additional component, the model is referred to as the Theory of Planned Action.

The Theory of Reasoned Action/Planned Behavior is similar, in many respects, to the Problem Behavior Theory. For example, the social psychological variable Jessor[45] called the Personality System includes the individuals' attitudes, beliefs, expectations, and outcomes of engaging in problem behaviors, as does the attitudinal component of the Theory of Reasoned Action. However, the Problem Behavior Theory focuses on more general attitudes. The subjective norm of the Theory of Reasoned Action/ Planned Behavior and Jessor's Perceived Environment System both include social norms and relationships among peer and parental influences.

The Theory of Reasoned Action has been used to predict successfully a variety of intentions and behaviors related to the issues of adolescent drinking and traffic safety. Budd and Spencer[54] used it to predict undergraduates' intentions to consume alcohol. They found that both attitudes toward the behavior and subjective norms were significantly related to intentions to drink. Furthermore, the weighted sum of attitudes and subjective norm was significantly predictive of intentions to drink.

This theory has also been employed in the field of traffic safety to predict intentions of use and actual use of safety belts[55] and to identify variables that are predictive of adolescent drinking and driving behaviors.[56–58] The Rothengatter and Jansen[56] results indicated that, with regard to the model, the main differences between drinkers and nondrinkers in the sample concerned the *beliefs about negative consequences* and their *evaluations of positive consequences* in social life. They further concluded that the differences between drinking drivers and nondrinking drivers concerned the *negative consequences of drinking,* and not, as one would suspect, the negative consequences of drinking and driving.

Sheehan and her colleagues[57,58] reported differences between frequent and infrequent drinkers, between males and females, and between rural and urban students with regard to the determinants of the attitudinal and normative components of intention and behavior. They found that males and females held different beliefs regarding the likelihood they would use alternative behaviors to avoid riding with an impaired driver, with females more likely to use alternatives. More pronounced differences were found between frequent drinkers and nonfrequent drinkers, with frequent drinkers significantly less likely to use 9 of the 10 alternatives listed. In comparing urban and rural students, they found that rural students thought it more likely that members of their families and social networks would drink and drive than did urban students; and rural, more than urban, students believed there would be more positive outcomes from drinking and driving.

Results from the San Diego County study provided additional support for the Theory of Planned Behavior. Five hundred and thirty-three students

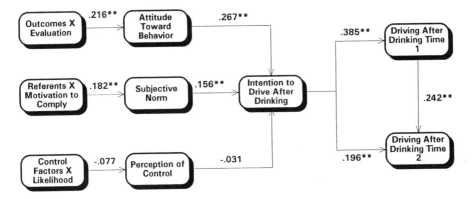

Fig. 1. Relationship of variables in model.

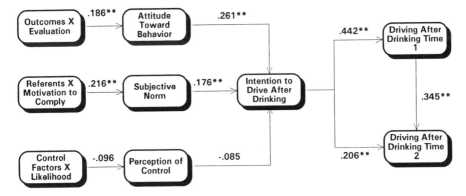

Fig. 2. Relationship of variables for drinkers only.

in grades 9–12 completed a battery of surveys that examined the determinants of the model. At 3 mo ($n = 500$) and 1 yr ($n = 417$) later, students were questioned regarding their drinking and driving behaviors. Figure 1 shows the relationships between the variables. As expected, intention was a strong predictor of behavior at both Time 1 and Time 2. Multiple regression analysis revealed that the components of the model taken together significantly predicted the intention to drive after drinking ($R = .281$, $p < .001$) and driving when over the legal limit at Time 1 ($R = .212$, $p < .001$), accounting for 8 and 4% of the variance, respectively. The components did not predict behavior at Time 2 ($R = .084$, $p > .10$).

The same analyses were conducted using only those students categorized as drinkers. The relationships of the variables are presented in Fig. 2.

As in the previous analysis, all expected relationships are significant with the exception of those involving the perception of control variables. Multiple regression analysis also yielded similar results with the components together predicting intention ($R = .283$, $p < .001$), accounting for 8% of the variance, and behavior at Time 1 ($R = .262$, $p < .001$), accounting for 7% of the variance. Again the components were not significantly predictive of behavior at Time 2.

Although providing partial support for the use of this model in the study of adolescent drinking and driving, a number of questions are raised by these findings. The component of perceived control was not at all related to intention as proposed by the model, making its contribution questionable. There are a number of possible explanations for this finding. First, Ajzen[53] suggested that this component was useful for those behaviors in which the individual has little or no volitional control. If this behavior does not fit that description, it is likely the component would have little added value. Second, it may be that the assessment of perception of control was not measuring the construct that was intended. The latter explanation seems plausible given that the determinants of this component were negatively related to the component. Further study of this portion of the model should be attempted.

Implications of the Theoretical Models

The importance of the theoretical models lie in their implications for interventions and prevention strategies. In understanding the predictors and correlates of adolescent drinking and driving and of alcohol-related crash involvement, we are in a better position to develop interventions and preventions that address the problem. Although policy changes have had some effect on reducing the incidence of adolescent deaths from alcohol-related motor vehicle crashes, development of strategies that focus on adolescent attitudes and normative pressures should have additional impact.

References

[1]E. C. Cerrelli (1992) *Crash Data and Rates for Age-Sex Groups of Drivers, 1990.* NHTSA DOT Research Note, May, Washington, DC.

[2]J. C. Fell (1987) *Alcohol Involvement Rates in Fatal Crashes: A Focus on Young Drivers and Female Drivers.* NHTSA Technical Report, DOT HS 807 184, Washington, DC.

[3]A. F. Williams and O. Carsten (1989) Driver age and crash involvement. *Am. J. Public Health* **79**, 326,327.

[4]National Highway Traffic Safety Administration (1988) *Fatal Accident Reporting System, 1986: A Review of Information of Fatal Traffic Accidents in the U.S. in*

1986. US Department of Transportation (Publication No. DOT-HS-807–245), Washington, DC.

[5]K. Stoddard and J. P. Rothe (1987) Young drivers: what has been written, in *Rethinking Young Drivers.* J. P. Rothe, ed. Insurance Corporation of British Columbia, Canada, pp. 5–13.

[6]D. R. Mayhew and H. M. Simpson (1985) Alcohol, age, and risk of road accident involvement.

[7]J. C. Fell and C. E. Nash (1989) The nature of the alcohol problem in U.S. fatal crashes, in *Alcohol, Drugs and Traffic Safety. Proceedings of the Ninth International Conference on Alcohol, Drugs and Traffic Safety, San Juan, Puerto Rico.* S. Kaye and G. W. Meier, eds. US Government Printing Office, No. 937-947, Washington, DC.

[8]T. L. Cameron (1982) Drinking and driving among American youth: beliefs and behaviors. *Drug Alcohol Depend.* **10,** 1–33.

[9]B. A. Jonah and N. E. Dawson (1987) Youth and risk: age differences in risky driving, risk perception, and risk utility. *Alcohol, Drugs, Driving* **3,** 13–29.

[10]M. Windle (1991) Alcohol use and abuse: some findings from the National Adolescent Student Health Survey. *Alcohol Health Res. World* **15,** 5–10.

[11]M. E. Fortini (1992) *Adolescent Drinking and Driving: Attitudes and Behaviors.* (Preliminary Report).

[12]R. A. Zucker and T. C. Harford (1983) National study of the demography of adolescent drinking practices in 1980. *J. Stud. Alcohol* **44,** 974–985.

[13]Health and Welfare Canada (1992) *National Survey on Drinking and Driving 1988.* Minister of Supply and Services Canada, Ottawa, Ontario.

[14]D. Elliott (1987) Self-reported driving while under the influence of alcohol/drugs and the risk of alcohol/drug related accidents. *Alcohol, Drugs, Driving* **3,** 31–43.

[15]Office of Technology Assessment (1990) *Adolescent Health.* US Congress, Washington, DC.

[16]California Department of Motor Vehicles (1993) *Annual Report of the California DUI Management Information System.* DMV Report, CAL-DMV-RSS-93-138, Sacramento.

[17]National Highway Traffic Safety Administration (1993) *Enforcement of Underage-Impaired Driving Laws: Issues, Problems, Recommended Solutions.* Department of Transportation (Publication No. DOT-HS-807–920), Washington, DC.

[18]M. E. Vegega and M. D. Klitzner (1989) Drinking and driving among youth: a study of situational risk factors. *Health Educ. Q.* **16,** 373–388.

[19]M. B. Roy, E. Greenblatt, and T. McDonagh (1979) Driving under the influence of liquor.

[20]L. P. Ivan (1984) Impact of head trauma on society. *Can. J. Neurol. Sci.* **11,** 417–420.

[21]L. Evans (1987) Young driver involvement in severe car crashes. *Alcohol, Drugs, Driving* **3,** 63–78.

[22]P. L. Zador (1991) Alcohol-related relative risk of fatal driver injuries in relation to driver age and sex. *J. Stud. Alcohol* **52,** 302–310.

[23]H. M. Simpson and D. R. Mayhew (1987) Demographic trends and traffic casualties among youth. *Alcohol, Drugs, Driving* **3,** 45–62.

[24]C. L. Popkin (1991) Drinking and driving by young females: recent trends in North Carolina. *Accident Anal. Prev.* **23,** 37–44.

[25]National Center for Statistics and Analysis (1991) *1991 Alcohol Fatal Crash Facts 1991 Traffic Fatality Facts.* US Department of Transportation—NHTSA, Washington, DC.

[26]R. D. Blomberg (1992) *Lower BAC Limits for Youth: Evaluation of the Maryland .02 Law.* NHTSA Technical Summary, US Department of Transportation (Publication No. DOT-HS-807–859), Washington, DC.

[27]N. E. Jones, C. F. Pieper, and L. S. Robertson (1992) Effect of legal drinking age on fatal injuries of adolescents and young adults. *Am. J. Public Health* **82,** 112–115.

[28]R. Hingson, T. Heeren, S. Morelock, and R. Lederman (1986) *Effects of Maine's .02 Law.* Presented at the International Symposium on Young Drivers' Alcohol and Drug Impairment, Amsterdam, The Netherlands.

[29]A. C. Wagenaar (1983) Raising the legal drinking age in Maine: impact on traffic accidents among young drivers. *Int. J. Addict.* **18,** 365–377.

[30]A. C. Wagenaar (1986) Preventing highway crashes by raising the legal minimum age for drinking: the Michigan experience 6 years later. *J. Safety Res.* **17,** 101–109.

[31]R. P. Lillis, T. P. Williams, and W. R.Williford (1984) *Impact of the 19 year old drinking age in New York.* National Alcoholism Forum, Detroit, MI.

[32]J. F. Mosher (1980) The history of youthful drinking laws: implications for current policy, in *Minimum-Drinking-Age Laws.* H. Weschler, ed. Lexington Books, Lexington, MA, pp. 11–38.

[33]R. P. Lillis, T. P. Williams, and W. R. Williford (1984) *Special Policy Considerations in Raising the Minimum Drinking Age: Border Crossing by Young Drivers.* National Alcoholism Forum, Detroit, MI.

[34]R. Hingson, J. Howland, S. Morelock, and T. Heeren (1988) Legal interventions to reduce drunken driving and related fatalities among youthful drivers. *Alcohol, Drugs, Driving* **4,** 87–98.

[35]R. Hingson, D. Merrigan, and T. Heeren (1985) Effects of Massachusetts raising its legal drinking age from 18 to 20 on deaths from teenage homicide, suicide, and nontraffic accidents. *Pediatr. Clin. N. Am.* **32,** 221–232.

[36]R. Zylman (1972) Drivers' records: are they a valid measure of driving behavior? *Accident Anal. Prev.* **4,** 333–349.

[37]National Transportation Safety Board (March 11, 1993) Letter to the Governors and Legislative Leaders of the States, the Commonwealth of Puerto Rico, the Territories, and to the Mayor of the District of Columbia. Safety Recommendation.

[38]J. F. Mosher (1985) Alcohol policy and the presidential commission on drunk driving: the paths not taken. *Accident Anal. Prev.* **17,** 239–250.

[39]B. C. Leigh (1989) Attitudes and expectancies as predictors of drinking habits: a comparison of three scales. *J. Stud. Alcohol* **50,** 432–440.

[40]B. C. Leigh (1987) Beliefs about the effects of alcohol on self and others. *J. Stud. Alcohol* **48,** 467–475.

[41]B. A. Christiansen, G. T. Smith, P. V. Roehling, and M. S. Goldman (1989) Using alcohol expectancies to predict adolescent drinking behavior after one year. *J. Consult. Clin. Psychol.* **57,** 93–99.

[42]D. L. McMillen, S. M. Smith, and E. Wells-Parker (1989) The effects of alcohol, expectancy, and sensation seeking on driving risk taking. *Addict. Behav.* **14,** 477–483.

[43]J. P. Rothe (ed.) (1987) *Rethinking young drivers.* Insurance Corporation of British Columbia, Canada.

[44]R. Jessor and S. L. Jessor (1977) *Problem Behavior and Psychosocial Development: A Longitudinal Study of Youth.* Academic, New York.

[45]R. Jessor (1987) Risky driving and adolescent problem behavior: an extension of Problem-Behavior Theory. *Alcohol, Drugs, Driving* **3**, 1–11.

[46]J. E. Donovan and R. Jessor (1978) Adolescent problem drinking: psychosocial correlates in a national sample study. *J. Stud. Alcohol* **39**, 1506–1524.

[47]R. Jessor, T. D. Graves, R. C. Hanson, and S. L. Jessor (1968) *Society, Personality, and Deviant Behavior: A Study of a Tri-Ethnic Community.* Holt, Rhinehart, & Winston, New York.

[48]R. Jessor, J. A. Chase, and J. E. Donovan (1980) Psychosocial correlates of marijuana use and problem drinking in a national sample of adolescents. *Am. J. Public Health* **70**, 604–613.

[49]D. J. Beirness and H. M. Simpson (1988) Lifestyle correlates of risky driving and accident involvement among youth. *Alcohol, Drugs, Driving* **4**, 193–204.

[50]V. Johnson and H. R. White (1989) An investigation of factors related to intoxicated driving behaviors among youth. *J. Stud. Alcohol* **50**, 320–330.

[51]I. Ajzen and M. Fishbein (1977) Attitude-behavior relations: a theoretical analysis and review of empirical research. *Psychol. Bull.* **84**, 888–918.

[52]I. Ajzen and M. Fishbein (1980) *Understanding Attitudes and Predicting Behavior.* Prentice-Hall, Englewood Cliffs, NJ.

[53]I. Ajzen (1985) From intentions to actions: a theory of planned behavior, in *Action-Control: From Cognition to Behavior.* J. Kuhl and J. Beckman, eds. Springer-Verlag, New York, pp. 11–40.

[54]R. J. Budd and C. P. Spencer (1986) Predicting undergraduates' intentions to drink. *J. Stud. Alcohol* **45**, 179–183.

[55]J. Wittenbraker, B. L. Gibbs, and L. R. Kahle (1983) Seat belt attitudes, habits, and behaviors: an adaptive amendment to the Fishbein model. *J. Appl. Soc. Psychol.* **45**, 326–333.

[56]J. A. Rothengatter and H. J. Jansen (1986) *Attitudes, Opinions, and Drinking-Driving Patterns of Young Drivers.* Proceedings of the 10th International Conference on Alcohol, Drugs and Traffic Safety, Amsterdam, The Netherlands.

[57]M. Sheehan, J. Majman, F. Schofield, V. Siskind, B. Smithurst, and R. Ballard (1986) *The Very Young Drink Driver: Defining the Problem for Prevention.* Proceedings of the 10th International Conference on Alcohol, Drugs and Traffic Safety, Amsterdam, The Netherlands.

[58]M. Sheehan, J. Majman, F. Schofield, V. Siskind, B. Smithurst, and R. Ballard (1986) *Social and Cultural Influences on Young Drink Drivers.* Proceedings of the 10th International Conference on Alcohol, Drugs and Traffic Safety, Amsterdam, The Netherlands.

Alcohol and Aviation Safety

Leonard E. Ross and Susan M. Ross

Introduction

Although the incidence of alcohol-related fatal aviation accidents has shown large decreases over the years and is far below the rate for highway vehicles, some pilots continue to fly while impaired by alcohol. A major safety study carried out by the National Transportation Safety Board (NTSB)[1] in 1984 examined fatal accidents during the period 1975–1981 and found no major air carrier accidents where the deceased pilot tested positive for alcohol, but did find that 6.4% of commuter airline, 7.4% of on-demand air taxi, and 10.5% of general aviation fatal accidents involved alcohol. This was a decline from the early 1960s when 30–40% of fatal aviation accidents were found to be alcohol positive.[2] A more recent NTSB report[3] shows a continuing reduction in alcohol-related fatal accidents. Through 1988 there still had not been a fatal scheduled commercial carrier accident in which the pilot tested positive for alcohol, no commuter airline fatal accident from 1982–1988 involved a positive-alcohol test of the pilot, and the alcohol-positive rate for on-demand air taxi accidents declined to 1.8%. General aviation fatal accidents during the 1982–1988 period had a 6.7% positive-alcohol rate. There is little evidence regarding the rate of alcohol involvement in nonfatal general aviation accidents since blood tests are rarely carried out in such situations.

The large decrease in fatal alcohol-related accidents that occurred after the 1960s was attributed to a pilot education program started in response to concern about the large number of alcohol-related fatal accidents previously experienced in aviation, as well as the introduction of Federal Aviation Administration (FAA) regulations prohibiting the use of alcohol by

From: *Drug and Alcohol Abuse Reviews, Vol. 7: Alcohol, Cocaine, and Accidents*
Ed.: R. R. Watson ©1995 Humana Press Inc., Totowa, NJ

crew members within 8 h of flight. The FAA adopted rules in 1985 and 1986 that prohibit persons from acting or attempting to act as a crew member while having .04% or more alcohol in the bloodstream, and provide for the suspension or revocation of pilot certificates for refusing to submit to a breath or other alcohol test or refusing to release the results of such a test.

The focus of the first section of this chapter is on recent studies of the effects of alcohol on pilot performance. Previous reviews of this topic[4,5] should be consulted for discussions of earlier studies and general issues relating to alcohol use in aviation. The second section is concerned with pilots' evaluation of various aspects of alcohol use in aviation and the factors that contribute to its use. Finally, issues that have been raised by recently enacted and proposed FAA rules are discussed.

Alcohol and Pilot Performance: General Considerations

It is commonly accepted that blood alcohol concentration (BAC) values above the FAA's .04% limit can degrade pilot performance and greatly increase the probability of an accident. Piloting an aircraft requires a variety of cognitive, attentional, and motor coordination processes that are known to be impaired by alcohol. Further, the increasing acceptance of the fact that automobile driving can be impaired by BAC values below .10% leads to the conclusion that pilot performance should be affected to a similar, if not greater, extent. For example, Moskowitz and Robinson[6] reviewed 177 studies concerned with alcohol effects on a wide range of skills and processes related to driving that would also be expected to be relevant to piloting an aircraft. Impairment was generally found at a BAC of .05% and appeared in many cases at values of .02–.03%. With respect to direct measurement of driver performance, some 8 of the 28 studies on this topic found impairment at BACs of .05%. If, as the authors concluded, BACs as low as .03% can produce significant impairment of driver performance and "no lower limit can be placed on alcohol impairment of driver-related skills," a similar impact of low BACs on pilot performance would be expected.

Not all studies have shown consistent alcohol effects on piloting tasks, however. This somewhat surprising fact must be interpreted in the light of several factors that can affect the relationship between BAC level and task performance, and thus complicate the problem of evaluating alcohol effects. The first is the nature of the experimental situation, especially the degree to which performance can be maintained if the individual's attention can be focused on a single task, albeit at the expense of other activities. Another related factor is the extent to which the subject can compensate with extra effort for the deleterious effects of alcohol. This is especially important when the effects of low BAC values are being investigated. Further complicating the situation is the fact that pilots differ in their competence level with respect to the various components of the flight task, and that alcohol's effects on the processes and skills involved may vary from individual to individual.

The manner in which the narrowing of attention can mitigate the effects of alcohol on some tasks at the expense of others can be seen in several studies. One of the most frequently cited articles on the topic of alcohol and pilot performance was reported in 1973 by Billings et al.[7] This study was carried out in an actual aircraft that had been instrumented to record the accuracy with which pilots could fly an instrument approach. The BAC values used in this study were 0, .04, .08, and .12%. The primary task required to fly the instrument approach accurately was to keep the two needles that indicated vertical and horizontal deviations from the desired approach path to landing centered. The pilots did surprisingly well in minimizing such flight path deviations while flying the glide path, even at the higher BAC values. They made significant numbers of serious major procedural errors during other segments of flight, however, such as failure to retract flaps before takeoff, flying at night without lights, and having the wrong radio settings, all of which reflected failure to distribute attention to the variety of tasks required in the cockpit. Overall, because of such errors, the safety pilot was required to avoid an accident by taking control of the aircraft 2, 4, and 16 times at the .04, .08, and .12% BAC values, respectively. Thus, although the pilots were able to compensate to a large degree in terms of focusing on the glide path task, their performance on other more distributed aspects of the situation was such as to create dangerous flight conditions.

Another important outcome of this study that should be mentioned was the demonstration that experience does not protect a pilot from the effects of alcohol. Although the highly experienced pilots made fewer major procedural errors than less experienced pilots, the rate of increase of such errors was identical for both experience levels. The 1984 NTSB report[1] also indicated that experienced pilots are susceptible to alcohol's effects. Twenty-six percent of pilots in alcohol-related fatal accidents had 1500 or more hours of flight time, and the flight-time group most over-represented in such accidents was the most experienced, i.e., those with 2500 or more flight hours.

The idea that alcohol can result in a focusing on one task at the expense of others is also supported by a study by Ross and Mundt,[8] which utilized an aircraft simulator instrumented to record a large number of flight performance measures simultaneously. It was found that even with low BAC values (mean of .043 and .038% at the beginning and end of the test sessions, respectively), subjects could do quite well in a navigation task that involved keeping a course deviation indicator centered, but they did so at the cost of altitude control where deviations were greater than those made under a placebo condition. Many individual performance measures in this study failed to show significant alcohol effects, although an overall performance measure based on a multiattribute model of flight performance did show a significant alcohol decrement.

These studies demonstrate that unless the flight situation requires distributed attention to component tasks, and performance on these components is measured, performance decrements owing to alcohol may be overlooked. A further complication in interpreting alcohol's effects on flight performance is the fact that individuals come into the flight situation with different component-task skill levels that may be differentially affected by alcohol. Yesavage et al.[9] pointed out that the high intersubject variability in subjects' responses to alcohol increases the possibility of false negative results because of increases in the variability of performance and the consequent reduction in the statistical power of the experiment to show alcohol effects. Greater response measure variability has been found in several studies of alcohol's effects on pilot performance.

With the exception of the Billings et al. study,[7] experiments investigating the effects of alcohol on pilot performance have used flight simulators. Simulators have been used for a variety of reasons, including:

1. The safety of the participants;
2. The relative costs involved;
3. The ability to control flight conditions so that they can be held constant from session to session;
4. The ability to introduce weather and aircraft systems problems and failures that could not be introduced safely in actual aircraft; and
5. The relative ease of obtaining quantitative measures of performance by interfacing computers to flight controls and instruments.

The major disadvantage of simulator use is the possibility that the data obtained may not accurately indicate the effects of alcohol in actual flight situations. For example, fatigue, anxiety, and stress levels may differ in the two situations, and simulators do not duplicate the sustained motion and g forces of actual flight that affect the visual–vestibular orientation system, which may be particularly sensitive to alcohol.[10] Pilots generally do take simulator flight quite seriously, however, and become very involved in the flight task.

It should be noted that there has been relatively little attempt to predict alcohol's effects on pilot performance from studies of alcohol's effects on laboratory tasks that are not analogs of flight tasks, e.g., laboratory studies employing experimental paradigms that presumably reflect cognitive or attentional processes. This reflects skepticism that more abstract process-oriented research, at least at the present time, can be generalized to the more complicated flying task. Indeed there is a lack of data demonstrating a predictive relationship between laboratory process task performance and flight performance.

Finally, although a detailed examination of the general methodological issues involved in alcohol research is beyond the scope of this chapter, there are a number of such factors that pose problems for research on pilot performance. These include task difficulty (ceiling and floor effects), the variability of subjects' ability levels, subjects' beliefs concerning the manner in which they are affected by alcohol, the success of double-blind procedures, and differing subject experience with the alcohol levels used.

Recent Studies
of Alcohol's Effects
on Pilot Performance

Recent studies of the effects of alcohol on pilot performance have generally investigated BAC values of .04% or below, or included such values in a range of BAC levels. Interest in BACs of .04% and below reflects acceptance of the fact that serious safety problems occur with BACs above that value, and interest in the adequacy of the FAA's .04% regulatory limit. Studies that have employed higher values usually do so in an effort to determine which aspects of flight are particularly impacted by alcohol, or the extent to which higher BAC levels interact with subject characteristics such as age. Studies reported in recent years employing a single BAC value in the .04% range or below include those by Davenport and Harris,[11] Ross et al.,[12] and Ross and Mundt,[8] the last of which was previously discussed.

Davenport and Harris[11] studied the flight performance of eight experienced pilots during visual and instrument approaches and landings in a simulator with the characteristics of a light twin-engined aircraft. Although .04% was the target BAC, the actual average BAC obtained was .011%. Despite this quite low BAC value, under alcohol conditions the eight subjects showed significantly larger lateral deviations from the desired horizontal glide path during instrument approaches, with larger deviations under conditions where one engine was inoperative. Very few procedural errors were noted. The authors suggest that the results demonstrate an alcohol decrement that is greatest under the most demanding cognitive work-load conditions. The fact that vertical deviations from the desired glide path did not show an overall alcohol effect was interpreted as "task shedding" where some tasks are maintained at the expense of others. It should also be noted that the standard deviations of vertical and horizontal deviation scores were many times as great with alcohol as with placebo conditions, although no statistical tests of these differences were reported.

Four experiments comparing pilots' simulator flight performance under low BAC (<.04%) and placebo conditions were reported by Ross et al.[12] Overall, the mean BACs of subjects when they started and finished the test sessions were .037 and .028%, respectively. Two of the experiments, one with 12 and one with 8 subjects, required the performance of demanding flight tasks under instrument meteorological conditions. The flight scenarios included complicated departure, holding, and approach procedures in one case, and navigation problems in the other. The other two experiments, with eight subjects each, involved instrument approaches under turbulence, cross wind, and simulated wind-shear conditions. In general, the first two experiments imposed relatively greater cognitive task loads on the subject, whereas the second two involved greater control-input task loads of a physical nature. Significant alcohol performance effects were found, but only during those parts of the flight scenarios that involved the greatest work load. In posttest interviews, 75% of the subjects reported mental or physical effects on their performance owing to alcohol, with a greater number of mental effects reports by subjects in the first two experiments and a greater number of physical effects reports by subjects in the second two experiments. A considerable number of the subjects reported that a greater effort was required to fly well after receiving alcohol. Thus, a large number of subjects reported the occurrence of mental or physical effects of alcohol, although performance decrements were found only under the most demanding flight situations. Apparently, subjects were able to compensate for alcohol effects on many of the flight tasks by expending extra effort. Such compensation, even at this low BAC level, could not prevent alcohol deficits when task difficulty became sufficiently great, however.

Turning to studies in which multiple BAC values have been employed, Billings et al.[13] carried out a study in which air carrier pilots were tested in a Boeing 727 simulator. This use of a jet aircraft simulator is in contrast to the usual procedure of testing general aviation pilots in a simulator representing relatively simple general aviation aircraft. Subjects flew eight simulated flights between San Francisco and Los Angeles with two flights at each of four target BAC levels; 0, .025, .050, and .075%. Records of cockpit activity were taken, with deviations from standardized procedures classified with respect to type and seriousness. Total errors made by the subjects increased with increasing BAC, with the major increase in errors found under the .075% BAC condition. Failures of vigilance, procedural, and performance errors all increased significantly, although crew coordination errors did not. Serious errors, defined as those with the potential to lead to loss of terrain separation, or warnings of such an event, did increase, but not significantly. Although both total and serious errors increased from the 0–.025% BAC conditions, only the serious error increase was significant. The reliability of this finding is questionable, however, given the fact that the .025% error rates were both higher in value than those found with a .05% BAC. It was also noted that alcohol effects were idiosyncratic with respect to the type of errors committed.

In another study involving multiple BAC values, Morrow et al.[14] tested pilots in a light aircraft simulator under various BAC conditions. This study used a different experimental procedure in that the pilot subjects flew seven flights during a single session at the times they attained a .04 and a .10% BAC, and then 2, 4, 8, 24, and 48 h after reaching the .10% BAC. In a separate placebo session, subjects flew at the same times following the start of the session that they had flown during the alcohol test session. Other features of this study included a comparison of two age groups of seven subjects each (mean ages of 25.3 and 42.1 yr) and an extensive examination of alcohol's effects on radio communications during the simulated flights. The flight scenarios were quite demanding, involving a series of changes in heading, altitude, communication frequency, and transponder settings during a six-legged pattern from takeoff to landing. System problems and engine malfunctions also increased the subjects' work load. A larger number of communication errors was found at the .10 than at the .04% BAC time points under both the alcohol and placebo conditions, although the difference was greater with alcohol. Significant impairment at the .10% BAC level was found only for older subjects, however. A significantly greater number of severe (100 ft or greater) altitude errors were made with alcohol than under the placebo condition. When tested at the .10% BAC value, older pilots made a greater number of such errors than young pilots. Off-course errors were greater with alcohol than under placebo conditions, and, although severe course errors were greater with alcohol, the difference was not statistically significant. When overall performance scores (combination of standardized scores for all performance measures) were analyzed, performance was found to be worse with alcohol than under placebo conditions, with the impairment still present 8 h after the subjects reached a .10% BAC.

As part of this study, the participating pilots rated their confidence in their ability to fly, their mood, alertness, and intoxication level before each flight. At the end of the flight, they rated the work load that the flight imposed and their performance. These rating data were interpreted by Morrow et al.[15] as showing that older pilots were more aware of their alcohol impairment and had less confidence in their flight performance after drinking alcohol than was the case for younger pilots. The younger pilots did not show awareness of their impairment except when tested 2 h after reaching a .10% BAC, although their confidence in their flying did decrease as alcohol impaired their performance. Surprisingly, in contrast to the verbal reports of subjects in other studies, ratings of work load did not vary significantly across the alcohol test conditions except that the older subjects rated flights as more difficult than did younger subjects. Subjects' mood scores showed an increase in positive mood as BAC increased, followed by a decrease with decreasing BAC. Thus, mood changes were inversely related to performance, with the highest mood scores associated with the poorest performance and mood scores decreasing with performance increases as BAC decreased over time.

Finally, a study by Morrow et al.[16] used procedures similar to those of the study by Morrow et al.[14] except that the subjects were not tested at a .04% BAC, the order of placebo and alcohol sessions was counterbalanced across subjects, and more hours of practice were given (8 vs 4). Two age groups of seven subjects each with mean ages of 25.8 and 37.9 yr were tested. In this study, performance was not related to the subject's age, and the effects of alcohol depended on the session order, with the alcohol impairment greater for subjects participating in the alcohol session first. A significant alcohol-placebo difference was found only at the .10% BAC, and 2 h later when the mean BAC had decreased to .071%. Performance was poorer after alcohol at the 4-h (.042% BAC) and 8-h (.002% BAC) tests, but the difference was not statistically significant. At each test point the subjects' performance variability was significantly greater under the alcohol conditions.

Pilots' Attitudes
Concerning Alcohol
and Aviation Safety

In order for educational programs and additional regulations to be effective in reducing alcohol use in aviation, it would appear that they should be developed with an understanding of pilots' knowledge, attitudes, and opinions about alcohol's effects. Such information is essential if educational programs are to provide the information that pilots need in order to make sound decisions about their own actions, and to ensure that regulatory efforts are seen as relevant and credible by the target population. Yet until fairly recently, little effort had been made to ask pilots for their views on topics concerning alcohol use in aviation.

The first effort to gather information directly from pilots was a regional survey carried out in 1978 by Damkot and Osga.[17] These authors sent questionnaires concerning drinking and flying to 835 Vermont pilots, approx 41% of whom responded. Three-quarters of the respondents indicated that it would be unsafe to attempt to pilot an aircraft within 1 h after drinking even one drink. Damkot and Osga also asked respondents to say how long a person should wait between drinking and attempting to fly. In spite of the "8-h rule," about half of the respondents indicated that it would be safe to fly within 4 h of drinking some alcohol, and the authors' estimates of the BACs, which would result under such circumstances, suggested that approx 30% of the respondents judged it safe to fly under conditions that could result in BACs of .015% or higher.

The first national survey of pilot attitudes toward alcohol use in aviation was carried out in 1988 by Ross and Ross.[18] In this survey, questionnaires concerning personal drinking habits and opinions about alcohol use prior to flying and driving were sent to a national sample of 2000 pilots. Sixty-three percent of the questionnaires were completed and returned. The questionnaire included a version of a drinking habits questionnaire developed by Cahalan et al.,[19] which made it possible to classify each respondent into one of five drinking categories ranging from abstainers to heavy drinkers. Respondents were very conservative in their attitudes toward the use of alcohol prior to flying as shown by their (median) judgment that it would not be safe to have even half of a drink 3 h before flying. For driving, however, their attitudes were quite different and were related to their individual drinking habits, with moderate and heavy drinkers much more tolerant of alcohol consumption prior to driving than were abstainers and infrequent drinkers.

In this survey, respondents were also asked to estimate the number of hours that a person should wait before flying or driving after having consumed various amounts of alcohol. The results showed a strong influence of the "8-h rule" in that even for as little as one or two drinks, median responses for individuals in all five categories of drinking habits indicated that at least 8 h should elapse between drinking and flying. Nevertheless, when estimated BACs were computed using the respondent's weight and the waiting interval they judged to be safe, 10–20% of the respondents would have had nonzero BACs if they had actually consumed the amount of alcohol in question and waited only the amount of time that they judged necessary to be safe before flying.

Although these two surveys are not completely comparable since one was regional and the other was based on a national sample, the results showed an encouraging trend over the decade; pilots in the more recent survey appeared to be more cautious about alcohol as compared to the respondents in the earlier survey. Nevertheless, pilots in both surveys estimated that it would be safe to fly under conditions such that alcohol would still be present in the bloodstream. This suggests that pilots may not have a good understanding of the relationship between the amount of alcohol consumed and the resulting BAC, and of the rate at which BAC decays over time. A second survey by Ross and Ross[20] addressed this topic. The questionnaire for this survey was sent to a national sample of 2000 licensed pilots, with 51.3% completed and returned. Many of the respondents' answers indicated that they did not understand the relationship between alcohol consumption and BAC. When they were asked to judge the BACs that would result from the consumption of various numbers of drinks, they consistently underestimated the consequent BAC, and when asked to judge how long it would take for BAC to decay to a safe level, they underestimated the necessary amount of time. These errors were more pronounced for moderate and heavy drinkers than for abstainers and infrequent drinkers.

This survey, carried out in 1987, also asked respondents if they were aware of the FAA's .04% BAC limit, which was established in 1985. Surprisingly, more than half of the respondents, including a majority of the flight instructors, reported that they had been unaware of the rule change prior to receiving the questionnaire. This finding and the finding that pilots do not understand how BAC is related to alcohol consumed or how it decreases over time highlight the need for more comprehensive educational programs concerning alcohol regulations and alcohol's effects.

A third survey by Ross and Ross[21] was sent to pilots holding the air transport pilot certificate, in order to obtain professional pilots' judgments about alcohol use in aviation. Over 60% of the 1000 pilots in the sample completed and returned their questionnaires. According to the respondents, alcohol use is more serious in general aviation than in corporate, charter, or airline activities. In response to several questions about the best way to reduce alcohol use in aviation, professional pilots expressed the opinion that greater enforcement efforts and harsher penalties are not likely to be effective. Instead, they endorsed approaches based on education and rehabilitation. In addition, respondents' comments suggested a number of social and environmental factors (e.g., home problems, economic concerns, scheduling, and various layover situations, such as limited rest time) that may contribute to the use of alcohol by professional pilots. The respondents indicated that pilots who cannot control their drinking are an important source of alcohol problems in aviation, with the key remedy being the effective functioning of employee assistance programs designed to encourage pilots with alcohol problems to seek help.

   In fact, inability to control alcohol use is seen by many to be a major factor contributing to alcohol use in aviation.[3] Alcohol dependence affects 7–10% of the US population, and it is estimated that the incidence of alcoholism is about the same for the pilot population. FAA regulations stipulate that a pilot who is an alcoholic may not receive a medical certificate. However, the regulations were amended in 1982 to permit alcohol-dependent pilots to apply for the special issuance of a medical certificate following rehabilitative treatment. This followed the passage of the Comprehensive Alcohol Abuse and Alcoholism Prevention, Treatment and Rehabilitation Act in 1970, as well as subsequent court tests of the act's applicability to medical evaluation of pilots and the FAA's reexamination of its medical certification standards. One of the main objectives of the 1970 legislation was to encourage alcohol-dependent individuals to seek treatment without fear of sanctions that would necessarily end their flying careers. Its success in this regard, at least for airline pilots, is evident in the fact that from 1960–1976, the FAA was notified of only 29 alcoholic pilots, 14 of whom were medically recertified, whereas 587 alcoholic airline pilots were granted special issuances of medical certificates after successful completion of a prescribed treatment program from 1972–1984.[22] By 1993, more than 1500 alcohol-dependent airline and corporate pilots had regained their medical certificates following rehabilitation.[23]

   The treatment regimen for alcoholic airline pilots was developed by the Air Line Pilots Association in cooperation with the FAA. It involves inpatient treatment, psychological evaluation, medical monitoring, and participation in aftercare programs such as those of Alcoholics Anonymous or Birds of a Feather. On completion of the treatment program, the pilot may apply for recertification. Followup studies of individuals who participated in rehabilitation programs and regained their medical certification have yielded very encouraging results in that 85–90% have been found to be still in good standing 2–5 yr later.[22,24,25] The success of treatment programs, both in terms of their ability to identify pilots who are alcohol-dependent and their ability to treat these individuals and return them to flight duties is, in large measure, the result of strong support at the corporate level and the high degree of motivation on the part of the participants.[22,23,26]

   Although the treatment approach is coercive in that the alcoholic pilot who wishes to keep flying must participate in the program in order to keep his or her flying credentials, it is directed specifically toward those individuals with drinking problems, and it offers the hope of rehabilitation and a return to flying. These features make it compatible with pilots' generally positive attitude about the effectiveness of this approach as a way to reduce alcohol problems in aviation[21] and help it gain pilots' support in identifying and reporting dangerous situations involving alcohol use. By reducing the number of pilots in the system who are high alcohol users, these programs also reduce the probability that dangerous withdrawal symptoms will occur during flight. Such withdrawal symptoms can occur when heavy drinkers cease drinking prior to reporting to duty after time off.[27]

FAA Rules and Issues

As previously mentioned, the FAA enacted rules in 1985 and 1986 that prohibit pilots from flying with a BAC at or above .04% and require pilots to submit to a breath or other alcohol test and release the results of such a test to the FAA. Criticisms of these regulations focus on two points. First, it is generally agreed that pilot performance can be impaired at BAC levels below .04%, and the possibility exists that setting such a limit may send a false message to pilots by suggesting that it is safe to fly with low alcohol levels. Also, the reported surveys demonstrate that if pilots attempt to predict their BAC levels from amount drunk or time since drinking, they are likely to seriously underestimate their BAC. The NTSB has consistently recommended that FAA regulations should prohibit individuals acting or attempting to act as a crew member when their BAC is at any value above zero. Second, although FAA regulations require reporting alcohol test results, few such tests are taken and no clear procedures exist for submitting, processing, and analyzing the tests that are taken. Law enforcement personnel often:

1. Are not at the scene of aviation accidents that do not result in fatalities or serous injuries;
2. May not be operating under implied consent provisions; and
3. May not have probable cause to require a test.

State laws vary widely with respect to these matters, and even if a test is taken there may not be a legal requirement that it be submitted to the FAA. Finally, the FAA appears not to have established procedures for receiving, processing, and analyzing state alcohol test reports once they are submitted to an FAA Flight Standards District Office.[3]

In 1990 the FAA introduced a program that used the National Driver Registry to screen medical certificate applicants for driving while intoxicated (DWI) offenses, and instituted regulations that require pilots to report DWI convictions or motor vehicle actions that involve any cancellation, suspension, revocation, or denial of a driver's license for any alcohol- or drug-related motor vehicle offense. Failure to report a DWI conviction or motor vehicle action is grounds for suspension or revocation of any pilot certificate or rating, or denial of an application for a certificate or rating for up to 1 yr. The occurrence of two or more alcohol- or drug-related motor vehicle actions within a 3-yr period can lead to the suspension or revocation of a pilot certificate.

Many pilots object to the DWI rules on the basis that one's driving behavior does not predict the driver's attitude toward drinking and flying and, more specifically, the probability that an individual will drink and fly. The FAA, in commenting on such objections to the proposed rule, admitted that they had made no attempt to obscure the lack of evidence that would indicate a correlation between drinking and driving and drinking and flying, but stated that convictions or administrative actions involving alcohol or drugs have relevance to such issues as pilots' judgment and their compliance disposition. There is no evidence of such generalized personality traits. The more commonly accepted and more plausible justification of the DWI rule, however, is that multiple DWI convictions, especially if based on high BAC values, have a reasonable probability of identifying a person with a serious drinking problem who cannot control his or her drinking and therefore is highly likely to drink and fly with a significant BAC.

In December 1992 the FAA published a notice of proposed rule making that would mandate random alcohol testing of flight crew member employees, attendants, flight instructors, and aircraft dispatchers; as well as those involved in aircraft maintenance, ground security, aviation screening, and air traffic control activities. This was in response to a congressional mandate (Public Law 102-143) that alcohol tests be carried out for all personnel engaged in safety sensitive commercial transportation operations. As proposed by the FAA, refusal to take a test, or a positive test result indicating a BAC of .04% or above, would result in immediate relief from safety-related responsibilities. Evaluation of the individual would follow, and, if deemed necessary, rehabilitation with followup testing would be required. In addition to random checks, tests would be conducted during preemployment screening, after an accident or incident, and on a followup basis after a failed test. If a random test revealed a BAC in the .02–04% range, a retest would be conducted 15 min later to see if the individual's BAC had fallen below .02%. If not, the person would be relieved of duty for 8 h.

There have been many criticisms of this proposal,[28] including objections to the presumption of guilt, the lack of cost effectiveness as demonstrated by the current drug testing results,[29] the lack of procedural safeguards for crew members being tested, and the failure of such tests to address the more serious problem of identifying the alcoholic problem drinker. Many see a greater payoff by directing resources toward enabling Air Medical

Examiners to identify the problem drinker and in strengthening employee assistance programs. At the present time the final form of this rule is not known.

A final issue is whether a regulatory approach will have the desired effect in the absence of educational programs designed to increase pilots' awareness of the danger of alcohol use in aviation. The reported surveys indicate that education is seen as important by pilots, and in its 1992 report[3] the NTSB strongly recommended that the FAA, in conjunction with various aviation organizations, develop new educational and informative material concerning alcohol and aviation safety, especially with a program emphasis on reaching the young pilot. Such material is seen as providing information concerning the effects of alcohol and other drugs on flying and their role in general aviation accidents, and as encouraging others to intervene when a pilot attempts to fly after drinking or using other drugs. To date there is little indication of educational efforts of this nature.

Acknowledgment

This chapter was prepared with the support of Grant AA-6093 from the National Institute on Alcohol Abuse and Alcoholism.

References

[1]National Transportation Safety Board (1984) *Safety Study: Statistical Review of Alcohol Involved Aviation Accidents*. NTSB Report No. NTSB/55/03, Washington, DC.

[2]L. C. Ryan and S. R. Mohler (1979) Current role of alcohol as a factor in civil aircraft accidents. *Aviat., Space, Environ. Med.* **50,** 275–279.

[3]National Transportation Safety Board (1992) *Safety Study: Alcohol and Other Drug Involvement in Fatal General Aviation Accidents, 1983 Through 1988*. NTSB Report No. NTSB/SS-92/03, Washington, DC.

[4]L. E. Ross and S. M. Ross (1985) Alcohol and drug use in aviation. *Alcohol Health Res. World* **9,** 34–41.

[5]J. G. Modell and J. M. Mountz (1990) Drinking and flying—the problem of alcohol use by pilots. *New Engl. J. Med.* **323,** 445–461.

[6]H. Moskowitz and C. D. Robinson (1988) *Effects of Low Doses of Alcohol on Driving-Related Skills: A Review of the Evidence*. DOT Report No. DOT/HS/807/280, US Department of Transportation, Washington, DC.

[7]C. E. Billings, R. L. Wick, R. J. Gerke, and R. C. Chase (1973) Effects of ethyl alcohol on pilot performance during instrument flight. *Aerospace Med.* **44,** 379–382.

[8]L. E. Ross and J. C. Mundt (1988) Multiattribute modeling analysis of the effects of a low blood alcohol level on pilot performance. *Hum. Factors* **39,** 293–304.

[9]J. Yesavage, J. Taylor, D. Morrow, and J. Tinklenberg (1992) The effects of alcohol on the variability of aircraft pilot performance. *Alcohol, Drugs, Driving* **8,** 217–224.

[10]H. L. Gibbons (1988) Alcohol, aviation, and safety revisited: a historical review and a suggestion. *Aviat., Space, Environ. Med.* **59,** 657–660.

[11]M. Davenport and D. Harris (1992) The effect of low blood alcohol levels on pilot performance in a series of simulated approach and landing trials. *Int. J. Aviat. Psychol.* **2,** 271–280.

[12]L. E. Ross, L. M. Yeazel, and A. W. Chau (1992) Pilot performance with blood alcohol concentrations below 0.04%. *Aviat., Space, Environ. Med.* **63,** 951–956.

[13]C. E. Billings, T. Demosthenes, T. R. White, and D. B. O'Hara (1991) Effects of alcohol on pilot performance in simulated flight. *Aviat., Space, Environ. Med.* **62,** 233–235.

[14]D. Morrow, V. Leirer, and J. Yesavage (1990) The influence of alcohol and aging on radio communication during flight. *Aviat., Space, Environ. Med.* **61,** 12–20.

[15]D. Morrow, V. Leirer, J. Yesavage, and J. Tinklenberg (1991) Alcohol, age, and piloting: judgment, mood, and actual performance. *Int. J. Addict.* **26,** 669–683.

[16]D. Morrow, J. Yesavage, V. Leirer, N. Dolhert, J. Taylor, and J. Tinklenberg (1993) The time-course of alcohol impairment of general aviation pilot performance in a Frasca 141 simulator. *Aviat., Space, Environ. Med.* **64,** 697–705.

[17]D. K. Damkot and G. A. Osga (1978) Survey of pilots' attitudes and opinions about drinking and flying. *Aviat., Space, Environ. Med.* **49,** 390–394.

[18]L. E. Ross and S. M. Ross (1988) Pilots' attitudes toward alcohol use and flying. *Aviat., Space, Environ. Med.* **59,** 913–919.

[19]D. Cahalan, I. H. Cisin, and N. M. Crossley (1969) *American Drinking Practices: A Study of Behavior and Attitudes.* Monograph No. 6, Rutgers Center for Alcohol Studies, Rutgers University, New Brunswick, NJ.

[20]S. M. Ross and L. E. Ross (1990) Pilots' knowledge of blood alcohol levels and the 0.04% blood alcohol concentration rule. *Aviat., Space, Environ. Med.* **61,** 412–417.

[21]L. E. Ross and S. M. Ross (1992) Professional pilots' evaluation of the extent, causes, and reduction of alcohol use in aviation. *Aviat., Space, Environ. Med.* **63,** 805–808.

[22]J. C. Russel and A. W. Davis (1985) *Alcohol Rehabilitation of Airline Pilots.* FAA/DOT Report No. DOT/FAA-AM-85-12, Federal Aviation Administration, Washington, DC.

[23]M. Gormley (1993) Help and hope for the alcoholic pilot. *Business Commercial Aviat.* **August,** 92–94.

[24]C. R. Harper (1983) Airline pilot alcoholism: one airline's experience. *Aviat., Space, Environ. Med.* **54,** 590,591.

[25]C. F. Flynn, M. S. Sturges, R. J. Swarsen, and G. M. Kohn (1993) Alcoholism and treatment in airline aviators: one company's results. *Aviat., Space, Environ. Med.* **64,** 314–318.

[26]R. W. Rigg, J. S. Storm, and J. Murdoch (1992) Industry drug and alcohol programs. *Aviat. Safety J.* **Spring,** 14–17.

[27]R. L. Wick (1992) Alcohol and pilot performance decrements. *Alcohol, Drugs, Driving* **8,** 207–215.

[28]S. L. Kalfus (1993) ALPA comments on proposed alcohol testing rules. *Air Line Pilot* **July,** 34–62.

[29]R. L. Wick (1993) Why pilot drug tests don't improve safety record. *Flying* **December,** 68–71.

Prevention Strategies for Reducing Alcohol Problems Including Alcohol-Related Trauma

Robert F. Saltz, Harold D. Holder, Joel W. Grube, Paul J. Gruenewald, and Robert B. Voas

Introduction

Drinking can increase the risk of injury and death depending on the activity or situation in which the drinkers find themselves. As a result, strategies to prevent or reduce the risk of alcohol-related trauma are best directed at drinking patterns or at drinking settings that involve risk or harm. The review of potential prevention strategies in this chapter identifies alternatives that have actually been implemented to reduce alcohol problems, whether they have been evaluated or not, and the available research evidence concerning the potential effectiveness of each strategy.

The traditional public health model of prevention identifies three elements of prevention: (1) the host, (2) the environment, and (3) the agent. Applying this simple model to the reduction of alcohol problems one is therefore concerned with

1. The individual drinker and his or her decisions and personal values about the use of alcohol;

From: *Drug and Alcohol Abuse Reviews, Vol. 7: Alcohol, Cocaine, and Accidents*
Ed.: R. R. Watson ©1995 Humana Press Inc., Totowa, NJ

2. The environment that surrounds the drinking context, including the drinking context and setting, the social group in which drinking takes place, and the physical environment in which drinking occurs;
3. The agent or the alcoholic beverage itself, defined as beer, wine, and distilled spirits alone or any mixture of these with other liquids such as fruit juice, milk, sweets, and so on.

This three-part public health model is used in this chapter to organize the overview of alternative prevention strategies, though in reality, interventions are often not easily categorized.

Policy Directed at the Individual

Alcohol policies directed at the individual are concerned with influencing personal decisions and values about drinking. Examples of such policies are education and communication to alter each drinker's decisions, and restrictions on advertising to reduce the promotion of beverages or the stimulation of alcohol sales.

Education and Communication

In the United States the largest investment of local, state, and federal prevention funds is directed at alcohol and drug education of young people in schools. This type of education is used not only for substance abuse but also for smoking and unsafe sexual activity among school-age young people. Moskowitz,[1] in a review of research through 1987, found that most such programs which were evaluated changed information and attitude levels but not self-reported alcohol and other drug use. More recently Pentz et al.,[2] from the evaluation of an extensive school-based educational program in Kansas City, MO, found reduced levels of alcohol- and drug-use initiation compared to schools without the program. More research is needed to demonstrate the effectiveness of the popular school-based education strategy in reducing actual consumption.

Public information campaigns have proven to be an effective means for soliciting community support for social interventions. For example, education, persuasion, and mobilization have been the main strategies to achieve women's right to vote, sales of war bonds, civil rights, and, more recently, cardiovascular disease risk reduction, and AIDS prevention.[3,4] Campaigns are typically considered along two dimensions: structural parameters and implementation processes. *Structural parameters* of campaigns are a set of purposive communication activities designed to reach a specified large audience over a specific period of time. *Implementation parameters* include:

1. Attention to underlying theory;[5,6]
2. Incorporation of formative research;[7]
3. Audience segmentation that allows targeting a specified audience; [8,9] and
4. Use of multiple channels of communication.[8]

Use of the mass media is also a popular means to encourage reduction of heavy drinking and/or drinking in high-risk situations, such as while driving. Moskowitz[1] (1989) concluded that there was no solid evidence that mass communication, by itself, has been successful in reducing drinking levels. However, the ability of mass communication in conjunction with small-group education and communication has been shown to be successful in reducing high-risk diet and smoking in a number of community trials for heart disease and cancer worldwide. (Some of these community prevention trials were reviewed by Giesbrecht et al.[10] and Farquhar and Fortmann.[11]

Worden et al.[12] conducted a public information campaign using "BAC Estimation" cards that provided data to drivers about steps to determine one's blood alcohol concentration (BAC). These "Know Your Limit" cards were widely distributed in an experimental community. Using roadside survey and community survey data, the authors found following the campaign only .06% of drivers in the experimental community were over the legal limit, whereas 3% of drivers were over the limit in the control community.

Following his review of public service information programs for the Surgeon General's Workshop on Drunk Driving, Atkin[13] concluded that:

> In general, mediated drunk-driving campaigns appear to have had relatively little effect on drinking and driving. This lack of significant influence is consistent with studies of related campaigns in the domains of safety belt promotion, substance abuse prevention, and other health practices. (p. 23)

Atkin[13] pointed out that there is increasing evidence of the potential for well-designed information campaigns to have behavioral effect using the principles of social marketing. This is especially true, according to Atkin, when formative research is used to develop campaigns that investigate the most effective sources, message appeals, and channels.

Vingilis and Coultes[14] reviewed the research evidence on mass media campaigns with other countermeasures, which they observed, comprise the majority of such purposeful communications programs. For example, mass information campaigns typically accompany the passage of new laws or specialized enforcement programs. They concluded from their review of such campaigns that the results were mixed, sometimes effects were achieved and sometimes not.

The major intervening factor between mass communications and drunk driving has been defined as the perceived risk of detection and/or apprehension for drunk driving, not the actual probability of arrest, which is quite low.[15-17]

Warning Labels

A recent public policy developed in the United States has mandated warning labels on alcoholic beverage containers. The required warning level in the United States is:

> **GOVERNMENT WARNING:** (1) According to the Surgeon General, women should not drink alcoholic beverages during pregnancy because of the risk of birth defects. (2) Consumption of alcoholic beverages impairs your ability to drive a car or operate machinery, and may cause health problems.

Warning labels are intended to lower risk associated with drinking while pregnant and/or while operating machinery. Hilton[18] reviewed existing research on warning labels. To be successful, people must read the warnings and thus be aware. If read, the content of the warning should be familiar. Greenfield et al.[19] conducted three waves of national telephone surveys during the survey months of 1989, 1990, and 1991. The results of these surveys showed that awareness of the warning label grew slowly over this time. Among respondents ages 18–29, the recognition ranged from 45–52%, among heavy drinkers (five or more drinks daily) the recognition was 50–59%, and among women ages 18–39 the recognition ranged from 35–42%.

The lower recognition among women in this childbearing age group was also observed by Hankin et al.[20] among Black, innercity pregnant women. Mazis et al.[21] found slow diffusion of the warning label in Gallup Polls from 1989 to 1991.

A recent report by Parker et al.[22] comparing pre- and postwarning label data found that drivers who drank and impaired drivers (based on self-reports) were more likely to recall the warning label and its content.

For the warning to reduce risk, people must be concerned about the content and actually change their drinking. Hankin et al.[23] found little increase in the perceived risk of drinking during pregnancy among pregnant women. The authors also found a 7-mo lag in the impact of the warning label on the drinking of pregnant women. There was a significant reduction in alcohol consumption among light drinkers but no change among pregnant heavy drinkers. This is similar to the conclusion of Parker et al.[22] who found no change in drinking and driving behavior among self-reported at-risk drinkers.

Greenfield et al.[19] found in their national survey that the proportion of people who reported deciding not to drive after "having too much to drink" rose from 35% in 1989 (prelabel) to 43% in 1990 (postlabel). Young males increased from 72–81% in their response to this question. Andrews et al.[24] found that college students found the drinking and driving warning to be believable.

Overall, the US alcohol container warning labels have achieved greater awareness over time, particularly among drinkers most at risk for alcohol-related problems noted in the warning. On the other hand, there is little evidence of behavioral change among those at-risk groups as a result of the warning label. However, there is evidence of increased cultural acceptance of the dangers associated with alcohol consumption as a result of the greater exposure to the warning labels in the general population.

Deterrence Approaches

An alternative rationale for public awareness has been developed in drinking and driving prevention. The primary basis for this approach is deterrence theory.[25–27] The theory states that the rate of crime (in this case, drinking and driving) varies with the certainty of detection and punishment. The key intervening variables between detection and punishment and the crime rate (driving while intoxicated [DWI] offenses) are the perceived probability of detection, severity of sanction, and the specific outcome measure (the BAC of drivers). The general validity of this theory in relation to alcohol safety laws has been demonstrated in a series of studies of naturally occurring variations in laws or in law enforcement recently reviewed by Ross[15] and Homel.[28] These studies also have demonstrated that of the two factors underlying deterrence, certainty of detection and severity of punishment, certainty of detection is the more important factor.[15,28,29]

Studies of legislative changes and enforcement programs make it clear that it is the perceived risk of apprehension not the actual probability of being arrested that determines the level of deterrence.[15–17] This finding has been confirmed by the research of Jonah and Wilson,[30] Vingilis and Salutin,[31] and Williams and Lund.[17] Because it is the perception rather than the reality of the detection risk that is significant to deterrence, some studies have found that drinking and driving can be manipulated through publicity alone.[31–34]

However, publicity alone has rarely produced lasting changes in safety behavior.[35] The best understanding of deterrence effects can be seen as an interaction between mass media information and the personal experience of drivers. Thus, Ross,[15] in his report on the British Road Safety Act of

1967, noted that the public was initially lead to believe that the probability of being tested for alcohol and arrested was much higher than it proved to be. He stated that, "It seems reasonable to me to ascribe (the subsequent reduction in effectiveness of the law) to the gradual learning by U.K. drivers that they had overestimated the certainty of punishment under the law" (p. 34).

An illustration of the interaction of publicity and enforcement is provided by the demonstration program sponsored by the National Highway Traffic Safety Administration (NHTSA) in Stockton, CA, which was evaluated by Voas and Hause.[36] A 7-yr trend in Friday and Saturday night accidents demonstrated that the addition of 10 extra police patrols dedicated to DWI enforcement (a 10-fold increase) on weekend evenings (which began on January 1, 1976) initially produced a large reduction in alcohol problems when the program attracted considerable coverage by local newspapers and electronic media. During this publicity phase, the crash rate declined by 25%. Later, when such coverage declined, the crash reduction was halved.

That the perception of risk is not dependent simply on the number of police officers devoted to DWI enforcement or the drinking driving laws is demonstrated by the "Cheshire Blitz" reported by Ross,[37] in which the impact of the of the Road Safety Act of 1967 in Britain was restored in one county by the constable ordering his officers to breath test all drivers in accidents or guilty of traffic infractions as provided by the law. This policy produced an immediate reduction in serious and fatal injuries but was abandoned by the constable after a month because of public pressure. A similar reduction in fatalities has been reported by Homel[28] following the adoption of an intensive breath testing program in Australia.

Although random testing received limited application in some countries in Europe with some success (in France, for example, as reported by Ross et al.[38]), most of the Australian states have implemented random testing as described by Homel.[28] In New South Wales, police were required to devote at least 1 h of each day to random breath testing of motorists. As a result, over a million breath tests were administered in a jurisdiction with 3 million drivers. This high rate of testing, together with a low *per se* BAC of 0.05%, has increased the perception of risk among Australian drinking drivers with the result that crash levels have dropped by as much as one-third in New South Wales and remained at this level for over 4 yr.[28,39]

Perceived Norms

One significant approach to reducing drinking and associated injury is to change perceived norms about drinking. Research consistently has shown that perceived norms or beliefs about the drinking behaviors of sig-

One type of alcohol ban has prevented distilled spirits from being sold in on-premise retail outlets. Although many monopoly countries control off-premise sales, on-premise sales have been largely private for some time. However, following the end of Prohibition in the United States, many states banned the on-premise sale of spirits. Holder and Blose[67] conducted an interrupted time-series analysis of counties within North Carolina, which first permitted such sales in 1968, compared with a comparison set of counties within the state that continued the ban. They found that spirits sales rose 6–7.4%. Associated with this increase in spirits consumption was a statistically significant increase in alcohol-related traffic crashes in these same counties.[68] This analysis used a multiple-level design intended to control for a number of threats to the validity of these conclusions. For example, traffic crashes involving drivers under 21 yr old who could not legally purchase spirits did not change, whereas crashes with drivers 21 and over did increase.

Density of Alcohol Outlets

The number and concentration of alcohol retail outlets are suggested to increase consumer convenience and possibly provide a social reinforcement of drinking behavior. Support for this observation has been provided by Colon,[69] Gliksman and Rush,[70] and Watts and Rabow.[71] Restrictions on alcohol availability through formal laws has been a central part of policy efforts in Canada and the United States as well in many other parts of the world.[72,73] Recent research conducted by Gruenewald et al.,[74,75] using two-stage least squares (2SLS) analyses and data from all 50 US states, found that outlet densities not only change in response to demand but also act to stimulate demand. As Gruenewald et al.[74] concluded:

> Greater sales of alcohol stimulated more alcohol outlets per capita....
> In a complimentary manner, increased license densities produced
> upward pressure upon alcohol beverage sales. (p. 18)

Price of Alcohol

Price has been an historically important part of prevention policy in many parts of the world. Alcoholic beverages appear to behave in the market like other goods, i.e., as prices decline and/or income increases, then alcohol consumption will tend to increase. A number of studies have estimated this relationship (the elasticity or sensitivity of alcohol consumption to changes in price and income).[76–79]

Grossman et al.[80] determined the differential price sensitivity of consumption by young people (16–21 yr old), paying special attention to beer, the alcoholic beverage of preference for the young. They concluded that youthful consumption is sensitive to price changes of both beer and distilled spirits and that increases in beer prices are not accompanied by increases in liquor and wine consumption. They found that a 10-cent increase in beer price will result in a 14.8% decrease in the number of youthful heavy beer drinkers (3–5 drinks of beer per day) and a 30-cent increase in the price of distilled spirits would result in a 27.3% decline in the number of youthful heavy liquor drinkers (3–5 drinks of liquor per day).

Since the overall consumption of distilled spirits as well as consumption of spirits by heavy drinkers can be demonstrated to be sensitive to price, it is reasonable to hypothesize that other alcohol-related problems will also be price sensitive. Cook[81] investigated the short-term effects of changes in liquor tax on the auto-accident death rates utilizing the same quasi-experimental design used to investigate the sensitivity of the correlation between liquor consumption and cirrhosis mortality. The same 39-state liquor tax changes used in the consumption study were employed. About 66% of the net-change observations for auto fatalities were negative. The probability that 66% or more would be negative is less than 4%. Therefore, one can conclude that a liquor tax increase tends to reduce the auto fatality rate.

Minimum Age of Purchase

There has been extensive research in the United States and Canada concerning the effects on alcohol problems among young people resulting from changes in the minimum age of purchase. This research has been summarized by Wagenaar,[82] Holder,[83] and the US General Accounting Office.[84] The US General Accounting Office concluded that there was solid scientific evidence that increasing the minimum age for purchasing alcohol has reduced the number of alcohol-related traffic crashes for young people under 21 yr old. A recent study by O'Malley and Wagenaar[85] found that a higher minimum-purchase age produced lower numbers of traffic crashes but also lower self-reported drinking. In addition, this preventative effect continues on as young people mature such that lower drinking levels and lower traffic problems involving alcohol can be observed even after young adults reach the legal age of purchase.

Server Intervention

An alternative intervention is at the primary location of drinking for impaired drivers. Studies of the location of drinking drivers have shown that substantial numbers of such drivers (in some cases the majority) are coming from licensed alcoholic beverage drinking establishments, i.e., pubs, bars, and restaurants.[86] These findings suggest that prevention interventions at such public drinking establishments could reduce the number of impaired drivers on the road. Mosher,[87] Saltz,[88,89] and others have discussed how changes in alcoholic beverage serving practices and establishment sale policies could be effective means in reducing the level of intoxication of customers, particularly those who subsequently drive. One means to accomplish such changes is to train servers in techniques to reduce the intoxication level of customers and to intervene in situations of high-risk drinking.

Servers can undertake a number of positive practices, including encouraging lower consumption by all consumers, but especially reducing heavy drinking. Servers can assist consumers in spacing their drinking out over time and increasing food consumption in order to slow down the absorption of alcohol. The effect of slowed alcohol absorption or increasing the length of time for alcohol absorption by the body can reduce the blood alcohol level (BAL) of the drinker and their level of impairment.

If the customer is intoxicated, the server can positively intervene by obtaining alternative transportation such as a taxi or nondrinking friends or relatives and/or by asking the customer to remain in the establishment until their BAL has reached a lower and potentially less impaired level.

Server training assists pubs, bars, and restaurants in changing serving and pricing policies to reduce the likelihood that customers will leave the establishment impaired. Reviews of the impact of server intervention on customers can be found in Saltz[90] and Gliksman and Single.[91]

In more recent research studies of server intervention, Saltz and Hennessy[92,93] and Saltz[94] demonstrated that such programs are most effective when coupled with a change in the serving and sales practices of the licensed establishment. Like the increased minimum drinking age, research into responsible beverage service has been used to support policies to encourage server training and prevention-oriented serving policies.

Evidence that changes in server practices can affect customer behavior comes from controlled evaluations of responsible beverage service programs. Changes in customer drinking behavior (lower number of high volume or intoxicated patrons) have been documented either through use of structured observations of customer consumption[88,89,95] or documentation of intervention with intoxicated customers using pseudo patrons (research assistants posing as customers)[91–93,96–98] as well as breathalyzer measures for pseudo patrons.[96]

Such research supports a conclusion that changes in server behavior can produce differences in the BAL of patrons leaving licensed establishments and thus the subsequent risk of becoming involved in a traffic crash or other alcohol-related problems. The results of this research were summarized by Saltz.[90]

However, such server training studies do not, by themselves, demonstrate that server intervention reduces alcohol-related traffic crashes or training given to a large number of servers can actually reduce aggregate levels of such crashes. The only state that mandates server training is Oregon. Utah encourages voluntary training but such training is not required.[99] One state, Texas, allows licensed establishments to obtain protection against liability suits if their serving employees have completed a state-approved training program.

The state of Oregon provides a unique opportunity to examine the research question whether server training provided to a significant percentage of all alcohol servers in a state can reduce alcohol-related traffic crashes. Prior to the mid-1980s, Oregon established a statewide requirement that all servers in retailed establishments selling alcohol must obtain permits. This permit was good for 5 yr. No special training was required to obtain this permit. In June 1987, the Oregon legislature passed state bill 726, which required that effective December 1, 1987, all new applicants for a beverage service permit must successfully complete a state-approved server training course. In addition, the bill required that all persons holding existing alcohol retail licenses or applying for new licenses must also complete a training program in 1987.

Holder and Wagenaar[100] conducted a time-series analysis of single-vehicle nighttime crashes in Oregon and demonstrated that when at least 50% of the servers of alcoholic beverages in a state and 100% of the licensees are trained, there is a statistically significant reduction in alcohol-related traffic crashes. A similar finding was obtained examining the effect of training for alcohol servers alone. This analysis has controlled for a number of alternative threats to this finding, including national trends in fatal crashes, which are strongly influenced by driving patterns and economic conditions. The effects of other significant traffic safety programs and legislation were also statistically controlled.

This finding, coupled with demonstrated ability of controlled evaluated server training to alter serving practices sufficiently to reduce the impairment level of customers leaving drinking establishments, strengthens the support for server training as a potentially effective means to reduce alcohol-related traffic problems. These results provide clear support for the potential of server training when completed by a significant percent (in this study, at least 40%) of all servers to reduce alcohol-related traffic crashes. This suggested that server training can be used effectively as a part of a comprehensive set of alcohol countermeasures.

Sanctions Against Service to Intoxicated Patrons

All US states have either criminal or civil sanctions against serving patrons who are obviously intoxicated. However, the effectiveness of these laws is a direct function of compliance and enforcement. Such compliance has rarely been studied. A recent study by McKnight[101] found that compliance, expressed as frequency of service intervention or termination, increased by 37% after visits and warnings by law enforcement. This was confirmed by a drop (from 31.2 to 24.6%) in the percentage of persons arrested for driving under the influence (DUI) who came from a bar or restaurant.

Server Liability

This liability is an indirect intervention into serving practices. It is based on a policy that alcohol-serving establishments are legally liable for the negative consequences caused by customers who were inappropriately served alcohol in their establishment. The prevention approach here is to encourage establishments to engage in safer alcohol-serving practices. This liability has been established in many US states following such situations as alcohol being served to an obviously intoxicated person who subsequently crashes his or her car and injures others or by serving to an underage drinker who is later involved in a trauma event.[99,102] The potential of such liability to bring about positive changes in the serving practices of retail establishments has not been comprehensively evaluated. A recent time-series study by Wagenaar and Holder[103] found that a sudden change in server liability in Texas produced a statistically significant 6–7% reduction in alcohol-related traffic crashes. Unfortunately, this macrolevel study was not able to directly document changes in server behavior in response to liability, and further replication of the study in other locations is necessary.

Restrictions on the Drinker's Behavior

These types of environmental policies directly or indirectly limit or restrict the behavior of the drinker or define the acceptable locations for drinking. Four examples of such policies are noted here:

1. Curfew laws;
2. Proscriptive and prescriptive norms;
3. Drinking and driving enforcement; and
4. Restrictions on drinking locations.

Curfew Laws

These laws establish a time when children and young people below certain ages must be home. Although this policy has not initially considered an alcohol-problem prevention strategy, research has shown positive effects. In those states that established such curfews, alcohol-related traffic crashes involving young people below the curfew age declined. (*See* research findings of Williams et al.[104] and Preusser et al.[105])

Proscriptive and Prescriptive Norms

Such norms address the types and amount of drinking that are considered to be publicly acceptable. Proscriptive norms are those that require either no drinking or no drinking in certain situations, such as while or before driving. The temperance movements built on social values in North America and Europe produced total Prohibition in many countries during the early part of the 20th century. Prescriptive norms can specify levels of drinking that are acceptable and provide rules about an acceptable drinking amount. Social norms about drinking influence levels of consumption. For example, it has been suggested that norms about drinking may account for the reduction in per capita alcohol consumption in the United States beginning in the early 1980s when there were no economic reasons for this reduction, i.e., prices declined, availability increased, and income increased in general. (*See* discussions in Treno et al.,[106] Room,[107] Linsky et al.,[108] Partanen,[109] and Johnson et al.[65,110])

Although not always a part of formal policy in every country, laws and regulations on alcohol availability as well as legal sanctions about unacceptable behavior, such as drinking and driving, do have potentially powerful influences and limitations on drinking behavior. An example of a most dramatic manifestation of changes in social norms about drinking has been worldwide public concern about drinking and driving. One form of this change in the United States was the grassroots movement of Mothers Against Drunk Driving (MADD). Originally formed as a support and action group for families of victims of drunk-driving crashes, MADD increasingly drew public attention to the problem of drinking and driving. This is illustrated by the substantial increase in news coverage in North America about drinking and driving in the 1980s.[111] Media attention to this issue reinforced the public concern and considerable legislative action was taken at the state and federal levels to strengthen enforcement and increase the penalties for impaired driving.

Drinking and Driving Laws

Public policy intended to reduce alcohol-related traffic crashes and the associated injuries and deaths is most represented in each country by laws concerning drinking and driving. Most developed countries have increased the penalties for drunk driving and their enforcement of such laws during the last decade. A considerable research base exists that documents the relative effectiveness of *per se* laws, administrative license revocation laws, drinking and driving enforcement, and sanctions or punishment.

Per se laws specify the blood alcohol level or concentration at which a driver is considered legally impaired, i.e., the level at which a driver can be arrested and charged with drinking and driving. The *per se* level has been declining in Europe, Australia, New Zealand, and North America. This reduction in the legal level of driver impairment has been associated with reduced crash levels.[15,112,113]

Administrative license revocation laws permit a police officer to seize a driving permit at the time of arrest if the driver is found to be over the limit. This type of law increases the probability that the offender will lose his or her driving privilege and has been shown to increase general deterrence of impaired driving as evidenced by reductions in alcohol-related crashes in states adopting such legislation.[112,114] Sanctions or punishment of a person convicted of drinking and driving has also increased in most countries. One type of punishment which has been shown to be effective as a specific deterrent in reducing repeated incidents of drinking and driving is license revocation.[115] The loss of one's driver's license has reduced the exposure of persons convicted of DUI to accidents and driving violations of all types.[115-117]

Restrictions on Drinking Locations

This policy has been employed in a number of forms throughout the world in terms of locations, days, and hours of sale. Such specification of locations where drinking cannot occur includes laws about public drinking and/or public intoxication, as well as those that may prohibit drinking in parks or recreational areas or at the workplace. Discussions about these types of interventions are contained in Giesbrecht and Douglas[118] and *Prevention File.*[119]

There are few studies of the direct effects of hours and days of sale. Such variables typically have been included as a part of multivariate analyses of variables related to alcohol consumption rates,[120,121] and in general measures of availability determined by formal laws.[122,123]

Smith[124] presented a study in which the introduction of Sunday alcohol sales in the city of Brisbane, Australia is related to casualty and reported property damage traffic crashes. Pre–post chi-square tests of problem rates aggregated over 2 yr before and 3 yr after the change in Sunday sales were used to test whether this change in availability had the expected impact. Estimates of the relative daily rates of problems were constructed by comparing Sunday rates to rates on other days of the week. Similar tests in surrounding comparison communities were used as controls for other possible contemporaneous changes affecting traffic crashes in the geographic area at large. Smith found that the measured relative daily rates did in fact increase in Brisbane, but not in the comparison communities, and that the time of day of these increases reflected the new opening hours of alcohol outlets. As he noted, the striking temporal relationships among these variables strongly suggests that hours and days of sale can have a substantial impact on alcohol problems. However, these results are not unequivocal as these effects could be contaminated by other trend effects on Sunday sales and nonequivalent distribution of crashes over days of the week.[125]

Olsson and Wikstrom[126] examined the effects of an experimental Saturday closing of liquor retail stores in Sweden. They found an 8% reduction in alcohol sales and a corresponding reduction in intoxicated persons and the number of police interventions in domestic disturbances. Nordlund[127] analyzed the effects of an experimental 1-yr Saturday closing in Norway for state stores. The findings were that the Saturday closings had little effect on overall consumption and that consumers adjusted to the closing by purchasing wine and spirits on other days or by purchasing beer. He did find that effects on heavy, problematic abusers were significant. The number of police reports of drunkenness and domestic problems on Saturdays and early Sundays decreased dramatically.

Environmental Approaches that Directly Reduce Risk or Problem Severity

Such public policy concerns those strategies that reduce the risk of harm to individuals who may already be impaired by alcohol. Examples of these strategies include driver restraints, automobile ignition interlocks, self-extinguishing cigarets, and low- or no-alcohol beverages.

Driver and Occupant Restraints

Such restraints include the provisions and use of driver and passenger seat belts and air bags. These devices have been shown to reduce the risk of injury and death for automobile occupants, including drivers who are involved in a traffic crash. Although reducing the incidence and severity of injuries to occupants of an automobile in which the driver is impaired by alcohol, it does not reduce the incidence of such crashes or the risk to nonoccupants. (*See* US Department of Transportation[128] and Williams et al.[129] for the safety effects of such restraints.)

Automobile Ignition Interlocks

These are devices that can check the blood alcohol concentration of the driver before he or she begins to drive. If the level is above zero or some other proscribed limit, the automobile cannot be started. This device has been discussed as a potential means to reduce all drinking and driving, but has been used in the United States primarily as a means to prevent a multiple drinking and driving offender from starting his or her auto after drinking.[130]

Self-Extinguishing Cigarets

Such cigarets are an example of a safety approach to reduce the likelihood of fire, for example, in bed. Research has shown that often persons are drinking and smoking and a fire is begun in bed or on a cloth-covered piece of furniture. Cigarets will not continue to burn if they are not regularly used by a smoker. Such cigarets are proposed as a means to reduce the chance of fires at home or in hotels.

Low- or No-Alcohol Beverages

The changing norms regarding heavy drinking and drinking and driving have increased public interest in alternative drinks and manufacturers have responded by creating low-alcohol versions of standard beverages, such as beer and wine. These beverages have attracted attention in recent years in many countries as a potential means to reduce levels of absolute alcohol consumed, and thus, associated levels of intoxication. These lower alcohol beverages have been often taxed at lower levels that produces lower prices in countries such as Sweden, Norway, and Finland where low-alcohol beer is sold in grocery stores rather than in state-monopoly retail stores. This lower taxation has been used in many Scandinavian countries to encourage production of three classes of beer of differing alcohol content and at least two classes of wine. (*See* Österberg[131] for a summary of these policies.) In a similar manner, responsible beverage service programs often include promotions of low- and no-alcohol beverages. It should be noted that a significant controversy exists over whether these low-alcohol beverages increase consumption by enticing nondrinkers to become alcohol consumers or whether they reduce consumption by lowering the amount of alcohol consumed by moderate to heavy drinkers.

Conclusion

The research reviewed here provides a scientific basis for considering a variety of prevention interventions based on the empirical evidence for their effectiveness in reducing alcohol-related injuries, and particularly traffic crashes. Although many of these alcohol policy alternatives have been shown to reduce alcohol-related traffic crashes, these policies are "broad brush," i.e., they impact both drivers and nondrivers. They are not always specifically targeted to the reduction of alcohol-impaired drivers.

Perhaps the best example of a policy that most directly affects drinking before driving is responsible serving practices and server training and server liability. If the BAC of patrons in bars and restaurants is lowered as a result of server intervention, then drinking and driving is the alcohol-related problem most likely to be impacted. Yet other alcohol problems can also be affected, i.e., violence, falls, burns, and so on, which result from alcohol impairment.

This suggests that efforts to prevent alcohol-related trauma may best be seen as part of a public health perspective on community safety in which drinking and driving plays a major part, but other nontraffic causes of death and injury related to alcohol impairment are also a part. This has two advantages. First, strategies such as alcohol regulation are seen as part of the total injury prevention effort, and second, a larger base of public support can be developed.

Environmental alcohol policies have particular advantages. First, as structural or environmental approaches, they are not dependent on persuasion and individual driver judgment. Second, they do not necessarily decay over time. For example, the impact of zoning restrictions on outlet density may be permanent, whereas the perceived risk of detection for DUI, which has been shown to be a powerful strategy for reducing events of alcohol-impaired driving, typically decays over time. Reducing alcohol outlet density would have more lasting effects. Third, many of the alcohol policy strategies have provided clear, scientific evidence that they can reduce alcohol-related traffic crashes. This provides a solid empirical basis for considering such strategies. Fourth, alcohol policy strategies can work synergistically with more conventional enforcement and judicial strategies. For example, retail establishments can be stimulated to participate in server training by DUI enforcement. In like manner, server intervention with customers can reinforce the preventative aspects of enforcement by reminding customers of their risk and the need to use restraint in their drinking.

Implications for Research

In many cases, the alcohol prevention policies reviewed in this chapter were not designed to specifically reduce alcohol-related injuries. For example, although traffic crash reduction was a useful measure of success for changes in the minimum drinking age, the reduction of drinking by young people was the primary target. Alcohol-related traffic crashes are a desired and a convenient indicator (with the availability of archival crash records with which to construct long time series).

There is clear evidence (as reviewed in this chapter) that strategies for alcohol problem prevention can affect alcohol-related injuries. This has been shown in such alcohol policy areas as the minimum drinking age, changes in alcohol availability, alcohol prices, and so on. Therefore, there are at least two major research opportunities in the next decade.

First, the challenge is to seek integration in injury reduction. For example, responsible beverage service (RBS) programs can reduce the level of intoxication of patrons leaving licensed beverage establishments. This means that not only are drinking and driving events reduced but it is likely that public drunkenness, alcohol-related violence, drinking and drownings, and so on, are also reduced. The random breath testing of motorists in Australia was shown to reduce fighting in pubs. Thus alcohol problem prevention research has much to gain and to offer alcohol-related traffic safety research.

Second, another important future research area is the synergism of alcohol-related injury prevention strategies. Future prevention research should examine the interaction and mutual reinforcement of programs such as DUI enforcement, limitation of alcohol sales to minors, the training and mobilization of parents, and underage drinking (*see* discussion by Holder[132]). To date, much of alcohol problem prevention research has been focused on determining the effectiveness of a single prevention strategy or counter-measure program. This is necessary to determine the efficacy of such programs. However, there is reason to hypothesize that the combined effect of two or more strategies can exceed the sum of the two as separate strategies owing to their mutual reinforcement.

The effects of increased DUI enforcement have been shown to decay after the driving public develops a more realistic assessment of their actual low likelihood of being detected for drinking and driving. Therefore, it is certainly possible that other strategies, such as educational or structural changes in alcohol availability, can serve to reinforce enforcement strategies. In short, a major challenge for the future in alcohol prevention research will be to develop strategies and research techniques that can examine the ability of multiple interacting strategies to reduce alcohol-related injuries.

Acknowledgments

Research and preparation of this chapter were supported, in part, by the National Institute on Alcohol Abuse and Alcoholism Research Center grant AA06282 to the Prevention Research Center, Pacific Institute for Research and Evaluation.

References

[1]J. Moskowitz (1989) The primary prevention of alcohol problems: a critical review of the research literature. *J. Stud. Alcohol* **50(1),** 54–88.

[2]M. A. Pentz, J. H. Dwyer, D. P. MacKinnon, B. R. Flay, W. B. Hansen, E. Y. Wang, and C. A. Johnson (1989) A multicommunity trial for primary prevention of adolescent drug abuse. *JAMA* **261(22),** 3259–3266.

[3]J. Farquhar, N. Maccoby, P. Wood, J. K. Alexander, H. Breitrose, B. W. Brown, Jr., et al. (1977) Community education for cardiovascular health. *Lancet* **1,** 1192–1195.

[4]J. W. Farquhar, S. P. Fortmann, J. A. Flora, C. B. Taylor, W. L. Haskell, P. T. Williams, N. Maccoby, and P. D. Wood (1990) The Stanford five-city project: effects of community-wide education on cardiovascular disease risk factors. *JAMA* **264,** 359–365.

[5]J. W. Farquhar, N. Maccoby, and P. D. Wood (1985) Education and community studies, in *Oxford Textbook of Public Health,* vol. 3. W. W. Holland, R. Detels, and G. Knox, eds. Oxford University Press, Oxford, London, pp. 207–221.

[6]W. McGuire (1981) Theoretical foundations of campaigns, in *Public Communication Campaigns.* R. Rice and W. Paisley, eds. Sage, Beverly Hills, pp. 41–70.

[7]C. Atkin and V. Freimuth (1989) Formative evaluation research in campaign development, in *Public Communication Campaigns.* R. Rice and C. Atkin, eds. Sage, Beverly Hills, pp. 131–150.

[8]J. A. Flora, E. W. Maibach, and N. Maccoby (1989) The role of media across four levels of health promotion intervention. *Annu. Rev. Public Health* **10,** 181–201.

[9]M. D. Slater and J. A. Flora (1991) Health lifestyles: audience segmentation analysis for public health interventions. *Health Educ. Q.* **18(2),** 221–223.

[10]N. Giesbrecht, B. K. Hyndman, D. R. Bernardi, N. Coston, R. R. Douglas, R. G. Ferrence, et al. (1991) *Community Action Research Projects: Integrating Community Interests and Research Agenda in Multicomponent Initiatives.* Presented at the 36th International Institute on the Prevention and Treatment of Alcoholism, June 2–7, Stockholm, Sweden.

[11]J. Farquhar and S. Fortmann (1992) Phases for developing community trials: lessons for control of alcohol problems from research in cardiovascular disease, cancer, and adolescent health, in *Community Prevention Trials for Alcohol Problems: Methodological Issues.* H. Holder and J. Howard, eds. Praeger, Westport, CT, pp. 59–75.

[12]J. K. Worden, B. S. Flynn, D. G. Merrill, J. A. Waller, and L. D. Haugh (1989) Preventing alcohol-impaired driving through community self-regulation training. *Am. J. Public Health* **79(3),** 287–290.

[13]C. K. Atkin (1988) Mass communications effects on drinking and driving, in *Surgeon General's Workshop on Drunk Driving: Background Papers.* U.S. Department of Health and Human Services, Rockville, MD, pp. 15–34.

[14]E. Vingilis and B. Coultes (1990) Mass communications and drinking-driving: theories, practices and results. *Alcohol, Drugs, Driving* **6(2),** 61–81.

[15]H. L. Ross (1982) *Deterring the Drinking Driver: Legal Policy and Social Control,* Heath, Lexington, MA.

[16]R. B. Voas (1982) Selective enforcement during prime-time drinking-driving hours: a proposal for increasing deterrence. *Abstr. Rev. Alcohol Driving* **3(10–12),** 3–14.

[17]A. F. Williams and A. K. Lund (1984) Deterrent effects of roadblocks on drinking and driving. *Traffic Safety Eval. Res. Rev.* **3**, 7–18.

[18]M. E. Hilton (1992) *Perspectives and Prospects in Warning Label Research.* Paper presented at the 18th Annual Alcohol Epidemiology Symposium, May 30–June 5, Toronto, Ontario, Canada.

[19]T. K. Greenfield, K. L. Graves, and L. A. Kaskutas (1992) *Do Alcohol Warning Labels Work? Research Findings.* Paper presented at Alcohol Policy VIII, National Association for Public Health Policy, March 25–27, Washington, DC.

[20]J. R. Hankin, J. J. Sloan, I. J. Firestone, J. W. Ager, R. J. Sokol, S. S. Martier, and J. Townsend (1993) The alcohol beverage warning label: when did knowledge increase? *Alcohol. Clin. Exp. Res.* **17**(2), 428–430.

[21]M. B. Mazis, L. A. Morris, and J. L. Swasy (1991) An evaluation of the alcohol warning label: initial survey results. *J. Public Policy Marketing* **10**, 229–241.

[22]R. N. Parker, R. F. Saltz, and M. Hennessy (1993) *The Impact of Alcohol Beverage Container Warning Labels on Alcohol-Impaired Drivers, Drinking Drivers, and the General Population.* American Sociological Association meeting, August, Miami, FL.

[23]J. R. Hankin, J. J. Sloan, I. J. Firestone, J. W. Ager, R. J. Sokol, and S. S. Martier (1993) A time series analysis of the impact of the alcohol warning label on antenatal drinking. *Alcohol. Clin. Exp. Res.* **17**(2), 284–289.

[24]J. C. Andrews, R. G. Netemeyer, and S. Durvasula (1991) Effects of consumption frequency on believability and attitudes toward alcohol warning labels. *J. Con. Affairs* **25**(2), 323–338.

[25]J. P. Gibbs (1975) *Crime, Punishment and Deterence.* E. Isevich, New York.

[26]D. Beyleveld (1979) Deterrence research as a basis for deterence policies. *Howard J. Penology Crime Prev.* **18**, 135–149.

[27]D. Beyleveld (1979) Identifying, explaining, and predicting deterence. *Br. J. Criminology* **19**, 205–224.

[28]R. Homel (1988) *Policing and Punishing the Drinking Driver: A Study of General and Specific Deterence.* Springer-Verlag, New York.

[29]J. Andenaes (1983) Prevention and deterrence—general and special, in *Alcohol, Drugs and Traffic Safety.* S. Kaye and G.W. Meier, eds. Proceedings of the Ninth International Conference on Alcohol, Drugs and Traffic Safety [DOT HS 806 814 (1985)]. U.S. Department of Transportation, Washington, DC, pp. 31–40.

[30]B. A. Jonah and R. J. Wilson (1983) Improving the effectiveness of drinking-driving enforcement through increased efficiency. *Accident Anal. Prev.* **15**(6), 463–481.

[31]E. Vingilis and L. Salutin (1980) A prevention programme for drinking driving. *Accident Anal. Prev.* **12**, 267–274.

[32]G. Mercer (1985) The relationship among driving while impaired charges, police drinking-driving checkpoint activity, media coverage, and alcohol-related casualty traffic accidents. *Accident Anal. Prev.* **17**(6), 467–474.

[33]C. B. Liban, E. Vingilis, and H. Blefgen (1985) *Drinking-Driving Countermeasure Review: The Canadian Experience.* Addiction Research Foundation, Toronto, Canada.

[34]J. Lacey, J. R. Steward, and L. M. Marchetti (1990) *An Assessment of the Effects of Implementing and Publicizing Administrative License Revocation for DWI in Nevada.* Final Report on NHTSA Contract DTNH22-84-C-07289, 51 pp, NTIS, Springfield, VA.

[35]C. J. S. Wilde, J. L'Haste, D. Sheppard, and G. Wind (1971) *Road Safety Campaigns: Design and Evaluation,* Organization for Economic Co-operation and Development, Paris, France.

[36]R. B. Voas and J. M. Hause (1987) Deterring the drinking driver: the Stockton experience. *Accident Anal. Prev.* **19(2)**, 81–90.

[37]H. L. Ross (1977) Deterrence regained: the Cheshire constabulary's breathaliser blitz. *J. Legal Stud.* **6**, 241–249.

[38]H. L. Ross, R. McCleary, and T. Epperlein (1982) Deterrence of drinking and driving in France: an evaluation of the law of July 12, 1978. *Law Soc. Rev.* **16(3)**, 345–374.

[39]R. Arthurson (1985) *Evaluation of Random Breath Testing.* Traffic Authority of New South Wales, Research Note RN 10/85. Sydney, Australia.

[40]J. W. Grube and M. Morgan (1986) *Smoking, Drinking and Other Drug Use among Dublin Post-Primary School Pupils.* Economic and Social Research Institute, Dublin, Ireland.

[41]D. B. Kandel (1980) Drug and drinking behavior among youth. *Annu. Rev. Soc.* **6**, 235–285.

[42]L. Chassin (1984) Adolescent substance use and abuse, in *Adolescent Behavior Disorders: Foundations and Contemporary Concerns.* P. Karoly and J. J. Steffan, eds. Lexington Books, Lexington, MA, pp. 99–152.

[43]W. Downs (1987) A panel study of normative structure, adolescent alcohol use, and peer alcohol use. *J. Stud. Alcohol* **48**, 167–175.

[44]J. W. Grube and M. Morgan (1990) *The Development and Maintenance of Smoking, Drinking and Other Drug Use Among Dublin Post-Primary School Pupils.* Economic and Social Research Institute, Dublin, Ireland.

[45]J. W. Grube and M. Morgan (1990) Attitude–normative belief interactions: contingent consistency effects in the prediction of adolescent smoking, drinking, and drug use. *Soc. Psychol. Q.* **53**, 329–339.

[46]M. D. Klitzner, M. E. Vegega, and P. Gruenewald (1988) An empirical examination of the assumptions underlying youth drinking/driving prevention programs. *Eval. Program Plan.* **11**, 219–235.

[47]L. Smith-Donals, M. Smith, and M. Klitzner (1985) *Baseline Results for the Site I Program School High School Drinking/Driving Survey.* Pacific Institute for Research and Evaluation, Bethesda, MD.

[48]M. S. Goodstadt (1986) Alcohol education research and practice: a logical analysis of the two realities. *J. Drug Educ.* **16**, 349–364.

[49]M. S. Goodstadt (1986) School-based drug education in North America: what is wrong? What can be done? *J. School Health* **56**, 278–281.

[50]R. H. Hopkins, A. L. Mauss, K. A. Kearney, and R. A. Weisheit (1988) Comprehensive evaluation of a model alcohol education curriculum. *J. Stud. Alcohol* **49(1)**, 38–50.

[51]A. Mauss, R. H. Hopkins, R. A. Weisheit, and K. A. Kearney (1988) The problematic prospects for prevention in the classroom: should alcohol education programs be expected to reduce drinking by youth? *J. Stud. Alcohol* **40**, 51–61.

[52]M. Klitzner, E. Bamberger, C. Rossiter, and P. J. Gruenewald (1994) A quasi-experimental evaluation of Students Against Drunk Driving. *Am. J. Drug Alcohol Abuse* **20(1)**, 57–74.

[53]D. B. Kandel (1985) On processes of peer influences in adolescent drug use: a developmental perspective. *Adv. Alcohol Subst. Abuse* **4**, 139–163.

[54]L. Chassin, C. C. Presson, S. J. Sherman, E. Corty, and R. W. Olvashavsky (1984) Predicting the onset of cigarette smoking in adolescents: a longitudinal study. *J. Appl. Soc. Psychol.* **14**, 224–243.

[55]B. R. Flay, J. J. D'Avernas, J. A. Best, M. W. Kersell, and K. B. Ryan (1983) Cigarette smoking: why young people do it and ways of preventing it, in *Pediatric and Adolescent Behavioral Medicine: Issues in Treatment*. P. J. McGrath and P. Firestone, eds. Springer, New York, pp. 132–183.

[56]S. Sussman, C. W. Dent, J. Mestol-Rauch, C. A. Johnson, W. B. Hansen, and B. R. Flay (1988) Adolescent non-smokers, triers, and regular smokers' estimates of cigarette smoking prevalence: when do overestimates occur and by whom? *J. Appl. Soc. Psychol.* **18,** 537–551.

[57]S. J. Sherman, C. C. Presson, L. Chassin, E. Corty, and R. Olshavsky (1983) The false consensus effect in estimates of smoking prevalence: underlying mechanisms, *Personality Soc. Psychol. Bull.* **9,** 197–207.

[58]J. W. Graham, C. A. Johnson, W. B. Hansen, B. R. Flay, and M. Gee (1990) Drug use prevention programs, gender and ethnicity: evaluation of three seventh-grade project SMART cohorts. *Prev. Med.* **19,** 305–313.

[59]W. B. Hansen and J. W. Graham (1991) Preventing alcohol, marijuana, and cigarette use among adolescents: peer pressure resistance training versus establishing conservative norms. *Prev. Med.* **20(3),** 414–430.

[60]W. B. Hansen, J. W. Graham, B. H. Wolkenstein, B. Z. Lundy, J. Pearson, B. R. Flay, and C. A. Johnson (1988) Differential impact of three alcohol prevention curricula on hypothesized mediating variables. *J. Drug Educ.* **18,** 143–153.

[61]P. L. Ellickson and R. M. Bell (1990) Drug prevention in junior high: a multi-site longitudinal test. *Science* **247,** 1299–1305.

[62]M. E. Vegega and M. D. Klitzner (1988) What have we learned about youth anti-drinking-driving programs? *Eval. Program Plan.* **11,** 203–217.

[63]Institute of Medicine (1989) *Prevention and Treatment of Alcohol Problems: Research Opportunities*. National Academy Press, Washington, DC.

[64]S.L. Becker, J. A. Burke, R. A. Arbogast, M. H. Naughton, I. Backman, and E. Spohn (1989) Community programs to enhance in-school anti-tobacco efforts. *Prev. Med.* **18,** 221–228.

[65]C. A. Johnson, M. A. Pentz, M. D. Weber, J. H. Dwyer, N. Baer, D. P. MacKinnon, W. B. Hansen, and B. R. Flay (1990) Relative effectiveness of comprehensive community programming for drug abuse prevention with high-risk and low-risk adolescents. *J. Consult. Clin. Psychol.* **58(4),** 447–456.

[66]C. L. Perry, K. Klepp, and J. M. Shultz (1988) Primary prevention of cardiovascular disease: communitywide strategies for youth. *J. Consult. Clin. Psychol.* **56(3),** 358–364.

[67]H. D. Holder and J. O. Blose (1987) Impact of changes in distilled spirits availability on apparent consumption: a time series analysis of liquor-by-the-drink. *Br. J. Addict.* **82,** 623–631.

[68]J. O. Blose and H. D. Holder (1987) Liquor-by-the-drink and alcohol-related traffic crashes: a natural experiment using time-series analysis. *J. Stud. Alcohol* **48,** 52–60.

[69]I. Colon (1982) The influence of state monopoly of alcohol distribution and the frequency of package stores on single motor vehicle fatalities. *Am. J. Drug Alcohol Abuse* **9,** 325–331.

[70]L. Gliksman and B. R. Rush (1986) Alcohol availability, alcohol consumption and alcohol related damage. II. The role of sociodemographic factors. *J. Stud. Alcohol* **47,** 11–18.

[71]R. K. Watts and J. Rabow (1983) Alcohol availability and alcohol-related problems in 213 California cities. *Alcohol. Clin. Exp. Res.* **7,** 47–58.

[72]R. Room (1987) *Alcohol Monopolies in the U.S.A.: Challenges and Opportunities.* Paper presented at a meeting on "The Role of Alcohol Monopolies," organized by the Swedish Systembolaget, January 20–22, Vaxholm, Sweden.

[73]T. Kortteinen (1989) *State Monopolies and Alcohol Prevention.* The Social Science Institute of Alcohol Studies, Helsinki, Report No. 181.

[74]P. J. Gruenewald, P. Madden, and K. Janes (1992) Alcohol availability and the formal power and resources of state alcohol beverage control agencies. *Alcohol. Clin. Exp. Res.* **16(3),** 591–597.

[75]P.J. Gruenewald, W. R. Ponicki, and H. D. Holder (1993) The relationship of outlet densities to alcohol consumption: a time series cross-sectional analysis. *Alcohol. Clin. Exp. Res.* **17(1),** 38–47.

[76]E. Österberg (1975) *The Pricing of Alcoholic Beverages as an Instrument of Control Policy.* Reports from the Social Research Institute on Alcohol Studies No. 83, Helsinki, Finland.

[77]H. Saffer and M. Grossman (1987) Beer taxes, the legal drinking age, and youth motor vehicle fatalities. *J. Legal Stud.* **16,** 351–374.

[78]D. Levy and N. Sheflin (1983) New evidence on controlling alcohol use through price. *J. Stud. Alcohol* **44,** 920–937.

[79]P. J. Cook and G. Tauchen (1982) The effect of liquor taxes on heavy drinking. *Bell J. Econ.* **13,** 379–390.

[80]M. Grossman, D. Coate, and G. M. Arluck (1987) Price sensitivity of alcoholic beverages in the United States: youth alcohol consumption, in *Control Issues in Alcohol Abuse Prevention: Strategies for States and Communities.* H. D. Holder, ed. JAI Press, Greenwich, CT, pp. 169–198.

[81]P. J. Cook (1981) The effect of liquor taxes on drinking, cirrhosis, and auto accidents, in *Alcohol and Public Policy: Beyond the Shadow of Prohibition.* M. H. Moore and D. R. Gerstein, eds. National Academy Press, Washington, DC, pp. 255–285.

[82]A. C. Wagenaar (1983) *Alcohol, Young Drivers, and Traffic Accidents: Effects of Minimum-Age Laws.* Heath, Lexington, MA.

[83]H. D. Holder, ed. (1987) *Advances in Substance Abuse: Behavioral and Biological Research (Supplement 1—Control Issues in Alcohol Abuse Prevention: Strategies for States and Communities).* JAI Press, Greenwich, CT.

[84]U.S. General Accounting Office (1987) *Drinking-Age Laws: An Evaluation Synthesis of Their Impact on Highway Safety.* U.S. Superintendent of Documents, Washington, DC.

[85]P. M. O'Malley and A. C. Wagenaar (1991) Effects of minimum drinking age laws on alcohol use, related behaviors and traffic crash involvement among American youth: 1976–1987. *J. Stud. Alcohol* **52,** 478–491.

[86]M. A. O'Donnell (1985) Research on drinking locations of alcohol-impaired drivers: implication for prevention policies. *J. Public Health Policy* **6,** 510–526.

[87]J. Mosher (1987) *Liquor Liability Law.* Matthew-Bender, New York.

[88]R. F. Saltz (1985) Server intervention: conceptual overviews and current developments. *Alcohol, Drugs, Driving: Abstr. Rev.* **1,** 1–14.

[89]R. F. Saltz (1987) The role of bars and restaurants in preventing alcohol-impaired driving: an evaluation of server intervention. *Eval. Health Professions* **10(1),** 5–27.

[90]R. F. Saltz (1989) Research needs and opportunities in server intervention programs. *Health Educ. Q.* **16(3)**, 429–438.

[91]L. Gliksman and E. Single (1988) *A Field Evaluation of a Server Intervention Program: Accommodating Reality.* Paper presented at the Canadian Evaluation Society Meetings, Montreal, Canada.

[92]R. F. Saltz and M. Hennessy (1990) *The Efficacy of "Responsible Beverage Service" Programs in Reducing Intoxication.* Prevention Research Center, Berkeley, CA.

[93]R. F. Saltz and M. Hennessy (1990) *Reducing Intoxication in Commercial Establishments: An Evaluation of Responsible Beverage Service Practices.* Prevention Research Center, Berkeley, CA.

[94]R. F. Saltz (1988) *Server Intervention and Responsible Beverage Service Programs.* Surgeon General's Workshop on Drunk Driving, Washington, DC.

[95]M. Hennessy and R. F. Saltz (1990) The situational riskiness of alcoholic beverages. *J. Stud. Alcohol* **51(5)**, 422–427.

[96]N. W. Russ and E. S. Geller (1987) Training bar personnel to prevent drunken driving: a field evaluation. *Am. J. Public Health* **77**, 952–954.

[97]E. S. Geller, N. W. Russ, and W. A. Delphos (1987) Does server intervention make a difference? *Alcohol Health Res. World* **11**, 64–69.

[98]A. J. McKnight (1987) *Development and Field Test of a Responsible Alcohol Service Program. Volume I: Research Findings.* National Highway Traffic Safety Administration, U.S. Department of Transportation, Report No. DOT HS 807 221.

[99]H. D. Holder, K. Janes, J. Mosher, R. Saltz, S. Spurr, and A. C. Wagenaar (1993) Alcoholic beverage server liability and the reduction of alcohol-involved problems. *J. Stud. Alcohol* **54(1)**, 232–236.

[100]H. D. Holder and A. C. Wagenaar (1994) Mandated server training and reduced alcohol-involved traffic crashes: a time series analysis of the Oregon experience. *Accident Anal. Prev.* **26(1)**, 89–97.

[101]J. McKnight (1992) *Enforcement and Server Intervention: Report to the National Highway Traffic Safety Administration.* The National Public Service Research Institute, Washington, DC.

[102]J. Mosher (1979) Dram shop liability and the prevention of alcohol-related problems. *J. Stud. Alcohol* **9**, 733–798.

[103]A. C. Wagenaar and H. D. Holder (1991) Effects of alcoholic beverage server liability on traffic crash injuries. *Alcohol. Clin. Exp. Res.* **15(6)**, 942–947.

[104]A. F. Williams, A. K. Lund, and D. F. Preusser (1984) *Night Driving Curfews in New York and Louisiana: Results of a Questionnaire Survey.* Insurance Institute for Highway Safety, Washington, DC.

[105]D. F. Preusser, A. F. Williams, P. L. Zador, and R. D. Blomberg (1984) The effect of curfew laws on motor vehicle crashes. *Law Policy* **6**, 115–128.

[106]A. J. Treno, R. N. Parker, and H. D. Holder (1993) Understanding U.S. alcohol consumption with cultural and economic factors: a multivarate series analysis, 1950–1986. *J. Stud. Alcohol* **54(2)**, 146–156.

[107]R. Room (1989) Cultural changes in drinking and trends in alcohol problem indicators: recent U.S. experience, in *Prevention and Control/Realities and Aspirations, vol. 3* (Proceedings of the 35th International Congress on Alcoholism and Drug Dependence). Ragnar Waahlberg, ed. National Directorate for the Prevention of Alcohol and Drug Problems, Oslo, Norway, pp. 820–831.

[108]A. S. Linsky, M. A. Strauss, and J. P. Colby, Jr. (1985) Stressful events, stressful conditions and alcohol problems in the United States: a partial test of Bale's theory. *J. Stud. Alcohol* **46,** 72–80.

[109]J. Partanen (1990) Alcohol in culture and social life. *Alcologia* **2(1),** 23–32.

[110]R. C. Johnson, C. T. Nagoshi, G. P. Danko, K. M. Honbo, and L. L. Chau (1990) Familial transmission of alcohol use norms and expectancies and reported alcohol use. *Alcohol. Clin. Exp. Res.* **14(2),** 216–220.

[111]J. D. McCarthy and D. S. Harvey (1989) Independent citizen advocacy: the past and the prospects, in *Surgeon General's Workshop on Drunk Driving: Background Papers.* U.S. Department of Health and Human Services, Washington, DC, pp. 247–260.

[112]P. Zador, A. Lund, M. Fields, and K. Weinberg (1989) Fatal crash involvement and laws against alcohol-impaired driving. *J. Public Health Policy* **10,** 467–485.

[113]C. B. Liban, E. R. Vingilis, and H. Blefgen (1987) The Canadian drinking-driving countermeasure experience. *Accident Anal. Prev.* **19(3),** 159–181.

[114]T. Klein (1989, July) *Changes in Alcohol-Involved Fatal Crashes Associated with Tougher State Alcohol Legislation.* National Highway Traffic Safety Administration, Washington, DC.

[115]R. Peck, D. Sadler, and M. Perrine (1985) The comparative effectiveness of alcohol rehabilitation and licensing control actions for drunk driving offenders: a review of the literature. *Alcohol, Drugs, Driving: Abstr. Rev.* **1(14),** 15–39.

[116]H. L. Ross (1991) *Administrative License Revocation for Drunk Drivers: Options and Choices in Three States.* Prepared for the AAA Foundation for Traffic Safety, April.

[117]A. J. McKnight and R. Voas (1991) The effect of license supervisor upon DWI recidivism. *Alcohol, Drugs, Driving* **7(1),** 43–54.

[118]N. Giesbrecht and R. R. Douglas (1990) *The Demonstration Project and Comprehensive Community Programming: Dilemmas in Preventing Alcohol-Related Problems.* Presented at the International Conference on Evaluating Community Prevention Strategies: Alcohol and Other Drugs, January 11–13, San Diego, CA.

[119]Communities mobilize to rescue the parks. (1991) *Prev. File* **6(1),** 7,8.

[120]J. F. Hoadley, B. C. Fuchs, and H. D. Holder (1984) The effect of alcohol beverage restrictions on consumption: a 25-year longitudinal analysis. *Am. J. Drug Alcohol Abuse* **10,** 375–401.

[121]J. P. Nelson (1988) *Effects of Regulation on Alcoholic Beverage Consumption: Regression Diagnostics and Influential Data.* Department of Economics, Pennsylvania State University, University Park, PA.

[122]R. G. Smart (1977) The relationship of availability of alcoholic beverages to per capita consumption and alcoholism rates. *J. Stud. Alcohol* **38,** 891–896.

[123]K. M. Janes and P. G. Gruenewald (1991) The role of formal law in alcohol control systems: a comparison among states. *Am. J. Drug Alcohol Abuse* **17(2),** 199–214.

[124]D. I. Smith (1988) Effect on traffic accidents of introducing Sunday alcohol sales in Brisbane, Australia. *Int. J. Addict.* **23,** 1091–1099.

[125]P. J. Gruenewald (1991) *Alcohol Problems and the Control of Availability: Theoretical and Empirical Issues.* Presented at the NIAAA conference Economic and Socioeconomic Issues in the Prevention of Alcohol-Related Problems, October 10–11, Bethesda, MD.

[126]O. Olsson and P.-O.H. Wikstrom (1982) Effects of the experimental Saturday closing of liquor retail stores in Sweden. *Contemp. Drug Problems* **XI(3),** 325–353.

[127]S. Nordlund (1985) *Effects of Saturday Closing of Wine and Spirits Shops in Norway.* Paper presented at the 31st International Institute on the Prevention and Treatment of Alcoholism, Rome, Italy, June 2–7. (National Institute for Alcohol Research, SIFA Mimeograph No. 5/85, Oslo.)

[128]U.S. Department of Transportation (1990) *Occupant Protection Facts.* Washington, DC.

[129]A. F. Williams, J. K. Wells, and A. K. Lund (1987) Shoulder belt use in four states with belt use laws. *Accident Anal. Prev.* **19(4),** 251–260.

[130]R. B. Voas (1988) Emerging technologies for controlling the drunk driver, in *Social Control of the Drunk Driver.* M. Laurence, J. Snortum, and F. Zimming, eds. The University of Chicago Press, Chicago, pp. 321–370.

[131]E. Österberg (1990) *Current Approaches to Limit Alcohol Abuse and the Negative Consequences of Use: A Comparative Overview of Available Options and an Assessment of Proven Effectiveness.* Presented at the Expert Meeting on the Negative Social Consequences of Alcohol Use, Oslo, Norway.

[132]H. D. Holder (1991) *Prevention of Alcohol-Related Accidents in the Community.* Presented at the International Symposium "Alcohol-Related Accidents and Injuries," Yverdon-les-Bains, Switzerland.

Alcohol as a Risk Factor for Drowning and Other Aquatic Injuries

Jonathan Howland, Thomas Mangione, Ralph Hingson, Gordon Smith, and Nicole Bell

Introduction

In 1991 there were 4600 drowning fatalities in the United States,[1] including 924 boating deaths.[2] For reasons that are unclear, drowning fatalities have decreased substantially over recent decades. Nevertheless, drowning remains the fourth most common cause of unintentional injury death for all ages and third for ages 5–44 yr.[1] Although the extent of morbidity related to aquatic activities is not fully known, the Centers for Disease Control and Prevention estimate that each year about 50,000 boating injuries are treated by emergency rooms;[3] the National Sporting Goods Association estimates that annually there are over 100,000 swimming injuries, 66,000 fishing injuries, 25,000 water skiing injuries, and 23,000 surfboard injuries requiring emergency room treatment.[1]

It is generally accepted among experts in aquatic safety that alcohol contributes to drowning rates. Indeed, there is increasing evidence to support this proposition in the form of studies of the prevalence of alcohol exposure among drowning victims and several case control studies (*see* Case Control Studies). Nevertheless, the causal role of alcohol in drowning is not entirely clear; it has not been demonstrated with the same quantity or

From: *Drug and Alcohol Abuse Reviews, Vol. 7: Alcohol, Cocaine, and Accidents*
Ed.: R. R. Watson ©1995 Humana Press Inc., Totowa, NJ

tity or quality of accumulated evidence as supports the association between drinking and increased risk for traffic injuries and fatalities.

The purpose of this chapter is to review what is known about the risks of drinking for untoward aquatic events, what is known generally about drinking behaviors on or near the water, and avenues for future research. Much of the research cited draws on the authors' work. Relevant studies by other investigators are discussed as available.

The Role of Alcohol

Alcohol Exposure Among Drowning Victims

Three literature reviews[4-6] on alcohol and nonvehicular injury have concluded that between 30 and 50% of adolescent and adult drownings had been drinking around the time of death. Over the past four decades there have been more than 40 studies published in the English language literature reporting on the proportion of series of drowning victims positive for alcohol on autopsy. Findings vary widely, from 15–86%. The wide variation in estimates result from different methods and from the fact that the majority of published studies are subject to potential bias owing to several design flaws common to most.

In many of the studies there was incomplete ascertainment of cases because only those in which alcohol use was suspected were tested. Most studies did not use—or make explicit—criteria for including or excluding cases based on duration of submergence. This is important because natural fermentation of decomposing tissue yields alcohol that can be mistaken for ingested beverage alcohol.[7] In some studies, exposure to alcohol is not determined by testing but rather on the basis of physical evidence at the scene (e.g., beer cans). In other studies, it is unclear which age groups are included in the denominator of drowning when the proportion exposed to alcohol is calculated. Since a large proportion of all drowning involves children under the age of 5, studies reporting on alcohol exposure among a series of drowning cases need to make clear whether very young children were included in the series. Alcohol is very rarely found in drowning victims under 15 years of age.

Nevertheless, several well-designed studies have been done controlling for these and other potential sources of bias. Waller[8] conducted a study of nonhighway injury fatalities occurring between 1965 and 1967 in Sacramento, CA. These included 17 submersion deaths meeting study criteria—cases submerged for less than 6 h. Of these, 29% were positive for alcohol. Dietz and Baker[9] reviewed alcohol involvement in drowning occurring in Baltimore and surrounding counties for the years 1968–1972. Only cases submerged less than 12 h were included. Of the 45 adult cases meeting study criteria, 47% were positive for alcohol. More recently, Berkelman[10] reported that 43% of 33 Georgia drownings were positive for alcohol, and Wintemute[11] found 41% of 234 drownings in Sacramento were positive for alcohol.

Alcohol Exposure Among Boating Fatalities

A 1990 review of the literature[12] on alcohol and boating fatalities reported on 16 published studies on the proportion of recreational boating fatalities positive for alcohol. Thirteen of these studies gave information on the proportion of boating fatalities exposed to any alcohol, and of these, nine also reported on the proportion with blood alcohol concentrations (BACs) in excess of .08. Three other studies reported only on the proportion with BACs greater than the statutory limit for the reporting area (BAC >.08 or >.10). Of the 13 studies reporting on any alcohol exposure among boating fatalities, percents exposed ranged from 7.5–82%, with little clustering. Of the 12 studies including data on BACs in excess of legal limits, proportions ranged from 14–64%, with 75% of studies reporting between 20–50% of fatalities with BACs in excess of statutory limits. The variations in exposure data underscores the need for careful studies—using consistent protocols—of drinking among boating fatalities, and aquatic fatalities in general.

Causal Pathways

The presumption that alcohol is a risk factor for drowning is plausible in several respects. Alcohol is known to be associated with physiological and cognitive effects that could contribute to drowning. For example, skills or judgment required to avoid life-threatening situations may be impaired among persons drinking in aquatic settings.[13] Alcohol affects balance and thus might precipitate falls into the water.[14] Alcohol creates a sensation of warmth that may lead some intoxicated swimmers to remain in cold water longer than if they had been sober.[15] At the same time, alcohol dilates blood vessels, thus increasing exposure of the blood supply to cold temperatures, and, accordingly, increasing risk for hypothermia. Alcohol may increase the risk for caloric labyrinthitis, an inner ear disturbance that could cause a person suddenly immersed in cold water to become disoriented and swim down rather than up.[15] Alcohol may also retard laryngospasm when water is aspirated, weaken the diving response, or inhibit response to asphyxial blood-gas changes (e.g., increased carbon dioxide levels).[16]

Field tests sponsored by the Coast Guard suggest that alcohol may work synergistically with environmental stressors (wind, glare, vibration, noise, and wave motion) to degrade performance of boaters. Results indicate that 4 h of exposure to boating stressors produced a kind of "boaters' hypnosis"—a fatigue affecting reaction times and course correction error rates similar to those caused by alcohol among car drivers.[17]

Case Control Studies

Most of the published studies on alcohol and drowning report the proportion of victims positive for alcohol. However, drinking is common among people engaging in aquatic activities and if there is no difference in alcohol exposure among drowning victims and noninjured individuals engaged in aquatic activities, alcohol's contribution to drowning is questionable. Accordingly, the argument for alcohol's causal role in drowning is enhanced when alcohol exposure data are also presented for noninjured controls matched on various characteristics thought to be related to the risks for drowning. This study design—the case control study—is the classic method for inferring causal associations in epidemiology. Few such case control studies have been conducted to measure risks for drowning in general or specifically the risks of alcohol for drowning. Two exceptions include a study currently underway of nonboating drownings in Maryland[18] and a study of California boating fatalities.[19]

Nonboating Fatalities

As part of an ongoing study of alcohol and drowning, one of the authors (Gordon Smith) is conducting a case control study on nonboating drownings in Maryland. This is the first case control study of drowning, and the first to specifically examine alcohol use among those who are exposed to water but not injured. BACs were collected on drowning fatalities by the medical examiner. Included in this study are those cases that occur in the daylight hours of the summer months from 1985–1993. Drowning victims had to be at least 10 yr of age. Preliminary results show a clear relationship between drinking and the likelihood of drowning: Drowning fatalities were as much as 32 times more likely to have been drinking than controls selected on the basis of age, gender, activity, and location of the drowning event. Indeed, even relatively low levels of blood alcohol (<.10) were shown to increase the risk of drowning fourfold. Although these results clearly are only preliminary, they potentially demonstrate a very strong causal role for alcohol in nonboat-related drownings.[18]

Boating Fatalities

There is also evidence that alcohol is a risk for boating fatalities. A 1988–1989 case control study was conducted on behalf of the Coast Guard to determine the estimated relative risk of drinking for boating deaths.[19] Information was collected on 57 California boating fatalities for whom good alcohol exposure data were available. This sample comprised 76% of all California boating fatalities for the years 1984 and 1985. Of these, 53% had zero BAC, whereas 34 and 21% had BACs greater or equal to .04 and .10, respectively. Investigators located boat ramps and marinas serving the bodies of water where the fatalities occurred and approached disembarking boaters (controls), requesting that they take a breath test. In all, 357 boaters were asked to participate, of which 92% complied. Forty-seven percent of fatalities vs 24% of controls had BACs greater than zero (odds ratio: 2.9). Twenty-one percent of fatalities vs 3% of controls had BACs >.10 (odds ratio: 10.6). These data may inflate the risk of drinking for boating fatalities because some disembarking boaters who had been drinking may have metabolized alcohol prior to landing. Moreover, the questionnaire used in the study collected little additional information and no information was obtained concerning cases' activities. Nevertheless, the magnitude of the risk derived from this study provides support for the view that drinking, and in particular heavy drinking, contributes to boating fatalities and injuries. Taken together with the preliminary findings from the Maryland drowning study, there is strong preliminary evidence that alcohol is an important risk factor for aquatic deaths.

Alcohol Use in Aquatic Settings

Frequency of Alcohol Use in Aquatic Settings

Alcohol use in aquatic settings is common. Results of a 1991 national household random digit-dial telephone survey conducted by Howland et al.[20] indicated that 89% of the population 16 yr of age and older reported at least one aquatic activity for the previous year. Forty-two percent of these respondents said they drank at least once before or during an aquatic activity during the year. When alcohol abstainers were eliminated from this analysis, 60% (70% of men and 51% of women) who drank at all (regardless of setting) and who had experienced an aquatic activity, drank on at least one aquatic outing during the year (Table 1).

Although many respondents said they drank at least once on or near the water during the previous year, the minority said they always or often drank in aquatic settings. Of respondents who said they drank in aquatic settings during the year, 9% said they "always" or "often" drank on or near the water, 36% said "sometimes," and 55% said "rarely."

This same survey queried respondents who said they had had an aquatic activity during the month before the interview about their last aquatic activity

Table 1
1991 National Aquatic Survey: Reported Alcohol Use in Aquatic Settings

Respondent group[a]	Percent			
	Total	Men	Women	p
During prior year				
All respondents with and without aquatic activities last year	38	48	29	<.00
Only respondents with aquatic activities last year	42	53	34	<.00
Only respondents with aquatic activities and who drank in any setting last year	60	70	51	<.00
Last day on/near water of last month				
All respondents with aquatic activity last year	28	33	23	<.00
Only respondents with aquatic activity last month who drank in any setting last year	37	42	33	<.00

[a]Age 16 or older.

day. Twenty-eight percent of these respondents (32% of men and 23% of women) said they drank alcohol on their last day on or near the water; men reported an average of 4.5 drinks on this day, women an average of 2.9 drinks. These data can be interpreted as the cross-sectional prevalence of alcohol exposure for a typical summer day in 1991 (Table 1).

Individuals' routine drinking behaviors were related to their propensity to drink in aquatic settings. Among those who drank at all during the year prior to the survey, heavier drinkers were more likely to report drinking in aquatic settings than lighter drinkers. About half the drinkers whose average daily volume of alcohol consumption was less than one drink said they had used alcohol on or near the water during the previous year. In contrast, 84% of respondents with average daily volumes of one to two drinks said they drank in aquatic settings during the previous year. Virtually all drinkers who reported an average of five or more drinks said they drank at least once on or near the water during the year prior to the survey (Fig. 1).

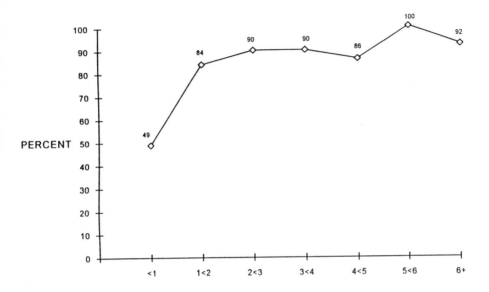

Fig. 1. Percent of drinkers who had aquatic activity last year and who drank at least once on/near water by average daily volume alcohol consumption.

Alcohol Use in Aquatic Settings by Age and Sex

The age and sex patterns of mortality rates for drowning are distinctive. For both sexes, rates peak between ages 1 and 2 and decline precipitously thereafter. Many of these younger deaths result from toddlers falling into residential pools and spas. Drowning rates for women remain very low through adolescent and adult years. In contrast, male drowning rates begin to increase in adolescent years, peak again in the late teens and early 20s, and then decline slowly but remain higher than women's rates throughout most of the adult years (Fig. 2).

This differential in drowning rates by sex and age suggests a number of hypotheses about differences in aquatic behaviors between the sexes. Evidence from our national survey indicated that adolescent and adult men on average spend more time on or near the water than women. Thus some portion of the drowning rate differential might be explained by differences in exposure to aquatic settings. Men may also be more likely than women to engage in risk-taking behaviors when on or near the water, although there is little published in the literature thus far to support this hypothesis. If alcohol were indeed a risk factor for drowning, then differences in alcohol use between men and women could also explain some of the differences in drowning rates by sex.

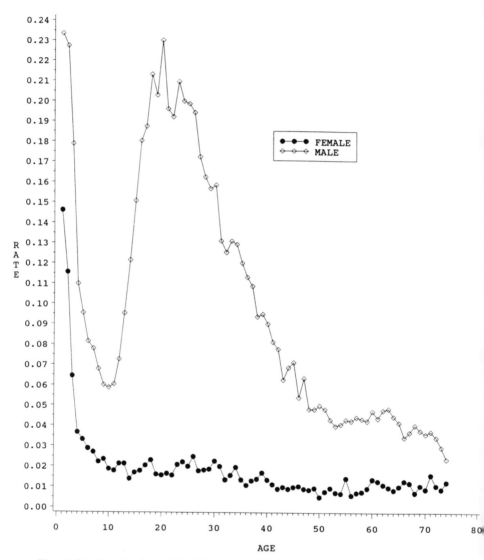

Fig. 2. Death rates (per 100,000) from drowning by age and sex for ages 0–75 from 1977–1979.

Our national aquatic activity survey demonstrated clear differences in alcohol use in aquatic settings by sex. Men were more apt than women to drink on or near the water for each 5-yr age group between 16 and 65 and for the age group 65+ yr (Fig. 3). This difference was smallest, however, for the age group 16–20 yr. Thirty-four percent and 30% of men and women,

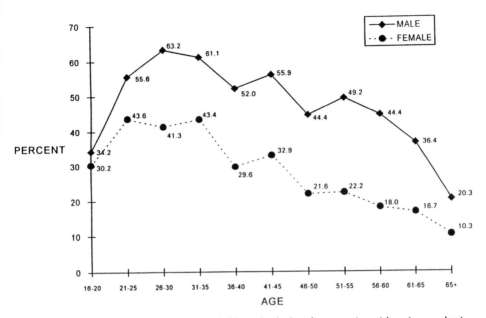

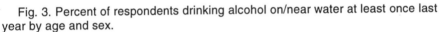

Fig. 3. Percent of respondents drinking alcohol on/near water at least once last year by age and sex.

respectively, in this age group said they drank on at least one occasion during the previous year. For men, the age group most likely to report drinking on or near the water was 26–30 yr. Sixty-three percent of male respondents in this age group said they drank on an aquatic outing at least once during the prior year. For women, the age groups most likely to report drinking on or near the water were 21–25 and 31–35 yr (44 and 43%, respectively). For both sexes, the likelihood of drinking in aquatic settings peaked between 20 and 30 yr of age and declined thereafter as the age of respondents increased.

Men not only were more likely than women to drink in aquatic settings, they also reported drinking a greater quantity of alcohol on a given outing. We compared men and women respondents to our national survey with respect to the amount of alcohol they reported drinking on their last aquatic activity day. Only respondents with an activity for the previous month were included in this analysis. Men, on average, drank more than women for each age group except 50–60 yr. The amount of alcohol tended to decrease with age for both sexes, with the mean number of drinks peaking for men and women in the 16–20 yr age group (Figs. 4 and 5).

In general, respondents said they drank a greater number of drinks in aquatic settings than they typically drank in other settings. This was par-

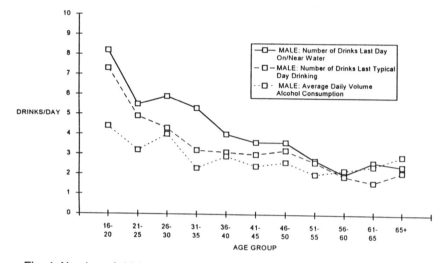

Fig. 4. Number of drinks last day on/near the water vs the number of drinks last day drinking vs average daily volume of alcohol consumption by age group for males who drank last day on/near water ($N = 302$).

ticularly true for men 25–35 yr of age, but the relationship held for most age-sex groups. For older men and women, there was a convergence between typical daily drinking and drinking in aquatic settings showing a gradual decline with age in the amount consumed in both settings.

Beverage of Choice

Beer was the alcoholic beverage most frequently cited as having been consumed in aquatic settings. Respondents to our national aquatic activity survey were asked what kind of drink or drinks they had had on their last day on or near the water. Of those who had used consumed alcohol, 70% said "beer," 21% said "wine" or "wine cooler," 16% said "hard liquor," and 3% said "some other alcoholic beverage."

Alcohol Use by Boaters

Although boating fatalities account for only 15–20% of aquatic deaths, there has been particular interest in alcohol's contribution to these events—in part, no doubt, because drinking and boating are seen as analogous to drinking and driving. Over the past two decades a number of studies[19-26] have been conducted to measure the frequency of drinking among boaters. Review of these studies suggests that between 25 and 50% of boaters drink when on their boats.[12] Variations in findings among these

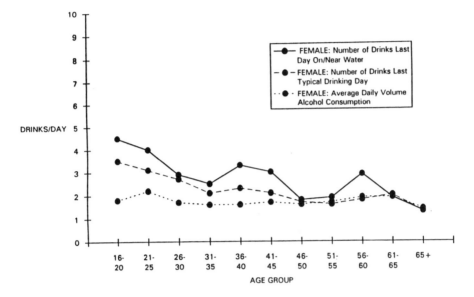

Fig. 5. Number of drinks last day on/near the water vs number of drinks last day drinking vs average daily volume of alcohol consumption by age group for females who drank last day on/near water ($N = 227$).

studies is probably owing to variations in when studies were conducted, methods used (e.g., dockside surveys, telephone interviews, mailed surveys), populations surveyed (e.g., boat club members, randomly selected households, and so on), and differences in the way in which alcohol use was operationalized.

Among those respondents to our survey who reported fishing from a boat, power boating, sailing, or water skiing during the previous year, 33, 32, 29, and 22%, respectively, said they drank alcohol on at least one of these outings. About 20% of individuals canoeing, kayaking, or rowing also said they drank on at least one outing in these types of boats. Thirteen percent of jet skiers and 12% of surf boarders reported using alcohol while jet skiing or surfing.[20]

When respondents were asked about their last day's boating experience, 21% of those who sailed, 20% of those who were on a power boat, and 17% of those who water skied said they used alcohol on that day. In contrast, only 9% of those who swam said they drank on their last aquatic activity day (Table 2). These results provide estimates of the prevalence of alcohol exposure during a typical summer day among persons engaged in these boating activities.[20]

Table 2
Alcohol Use Last Day On/Near Water of Previous Month[a]

Activity	N	Percent using alcohol
Sailing	30	21
Power boating	210	20
Water skiing	77	17
Swimming	1009	9
Jet skiing	24	4
Snorkeling/scuba diving	26	0

[a]By selected activity.

Alcohol's Enhancement of Aquatic Activities

A potentially important distinction between drinking and driving and drinking in aquatic settings is that typically one does not drink to enhance the driving experience; in contrast, drinking on or near the water combines two pleasures: drinking and aquatic activity. This difference may affect whether the public would be as willing to separate drinking in aquatic environments as they have been (over recent decades) in separating drinking and driving. To assess the degree to which persons who used alcohol on or near the water perceived drinking as enhancing their aquatic experience, surveyed respondents were asked about the pleasure enhancement of alcohol. Interestingly, 56% said that alcohol did not increase their enjoyment of being on or near the water at all and only 2% said that alcohol increased their enjoyment "very much," 18% said "somewhat," and 23% said "a little." These findings raise the question of why drinking on or near the water is so common and suggest that the demand for alcohol in aquatic settings may be subject to intervention.[20]

Intervention Strategies

Although the association between alcohol and drowning has been noted in the medical and public health literature for decades, interventions to reduce drinking on or near the water have been generally limited to boating. This is curious since only about 20% of drownings involve boats. For the most part, aquatic safety efforts have targeted skills training (e.g., Red Cross swimming lessons, Power Squadron boating instruction), behavioral issues other than drinking (swimming with a "buddy"), and environmental factors such as lifeguards, mandatory flotation for recreational boats, and regulations requiring life jackets on recreational boats.

Legal Strategies

There are currently no laws regulating the use of alcohol while engaging in nonboating aquatic activities. In some communities, there are laws prohibiting the use of alcohol on public beaches and these may affect the decision to use alcohol while swimming. They do not, however, specifically mandate that alcohol not be used by swimmers. There are laws restricting the use of alcohol while boating, perhaps because there is some precedent for this type of regulation drawn from regulation of motor vehicle driving. Nonboating alcohol regulations do not have a similar regulated activity from which to draw on for both public support and legal models or guidelines.

Our national survey of aquatic activities and associated drinking queried respondents about their support for laws controlling drinking in aquatic settings. When asked whether they would support or oppose laws prohibiting drinking at public swimming places in their communities, 63% of all respondents said they would "strongly" support such laws and another 22% said they would "somewhat" support such laws.[27] Similar support was shown for drinking and boating laws.[27] These data suggest that the public would support more aggressive local ordinances—or the enforcement thereof—targeting drinking in aquatic environments.

The Coast Guard Authorization Act of 1984 (Public Law 98-557) amended Title 46, United States Code, Chapter 23 (Operation of Vessels Generally) in two important ways. First, that portion of the Code dealing with negligent operation was expanded to include a section specific to operating a vessel while intoxicated. Second, the new section provided for the Secretary of Transportation to develop regulations prescribing standards for determining intoxication.

Subsequently, the Coast Guard established both a behavioral and a BAC standard (.10 for recreational boats). These laws apply to those bodies of water over which the Coast Guard has jurisdiction. By the beginning of the 1990s, 40 states had adopted similar legislation covering those waters falling under state and local jurisdiction and most other states had some version of drinking and boating laws. Nevertheless, there is considerable variation among these laws with respect to the way intoxication is operationalized and with respect to the severity of penalties.

Drinking and boating laws are difficult to enforce because the infrastructure for detecting and apprehending drunken boaters is not well developed. In contrast, drinking and driving laws are enforced by land-based police systems that were in place prior to increased efforts to deter drunken driving. Moreover, drinking and boating laws focus attention on boat operators as opposed to passengers despite the fact that almost half of boating fatalities involve boats that are not underway and only around 20% involve boat crashes. A third of boating fatalities involve falls overboard. A drinking passenger is at as much increased risk for drowning as the operator in most situations, and laws focusing only on drinking operators do not deter drinking by passengers.[28]

Nevertheless, the drinking and boating laws of the 1980s could have an important educational effect by underscoring the risks of alcohol use while boating. At present, however, results from our national aquatics survey indicate that only about a third of the adolescent and adult population are aware of the drinking and boating laws and fewer than half the people who said they were on recreational boats during the year prior to the interview said they knew about the these laws.[27]

Increased efforts to educate the public in general about the risks of drinking and boating (passengers as well as operators) and about legal sanctions for operating recreational boats while intoxicated should be a priority with the Coast Guard.

An informal survey we conducted of state boating law administrators suggests that Coast Guard resources for enforcement of drinking and boating laws are at a disadvantage with drug enforcement and search and rescue missions. Even when apprehensions are made, the federal judicial process is cumbersome and slow with regard to processing drinking and boating cases.

One method for increasing the effectiveness of drinking and boating laws has been adopted by several states.[29] In these states, boating violations involving alcohol are linked to motor vehicle licenses and become part of one's driving record. Other states should consider this approach as well. One state boating law official reported that about half the boaters apprehended for boating while intoxicated in his state in 1992 also had prior drunken driving citations (K. Elverum, personal communication, August 1993).

Another legal strategy for affecting drinking and boating would be to require licensing and/or mandatory training for boat operators. Removal of the license to operate a boat could provide an additional penalty for operating a boat while intoxicated. Mandatory training could provide an opportunity for informing boat operators about the risk to them—and their passengers—of drinking and boating.

There appears to be growing public support for these approaches.[26] Some states are adopting modified licensing laws requiring operator certification for targeted age groups or for motorized vessels over specified horsepowers. Other countries already have national laws requiring boat training and licensing, including Japan, Germany, and Greece.[29] Finland and Canada are also considering licensing laws.[29]

Another potential legal avenue for reducing alcohol-related boating mishaps would be the legal assignment, or partial assignment, of responsibility to the captain for the drinking behavior of crew and passengers. If the boat captain was held accountable for passenger safety in this way, he or she would probably be more mindful of the drinking behaviors of passengers. Also, many states have open container laws for motor vehicles. Similar laws might also be adopted for boats.

Educational Interventions

Organizations such as the Red Cross have been active for decades in promoting and conducting swimming lessons—particularly for children. These lessons include a variety of skill levels and swimming and lifesaving techniques. The net result of swimming lessons is, probably, an increase in exposure to aquatic environments, since nonswimmers may be less apt to go into the water intentionally. Indeed, many drowning victims are known to have been good swimmers. Moreover, the physiological effects of alcohol on individuals in the water may increase the risk of drowning regardless of swimming skills. Accordingly, information about the potential risk of using alcohol in aquatic settings should be incorporated into all swimming instruction programs—even for young children—and reinforced with public education.

A number of organizations have been established to promote boating safety. The most prominent of these include the Coast Guard Auxiliary, a volunteer organization established by a 1939 Congressional mandate; the US Power Squadrons, a private, nonprofit group established in 1914; and the National Association of State Boating Law Administrators, who administer and enforce state boating regulations.[29] There are many other organizations involved in boating safety, primarily through training.

Boating safety organizations and several beer companies have joined to promote a "designated boater" campaign similar to the "designated driver" efforts. Although this campaign may help to increase public awareness of the risks of drinking and boating, it may unintentionally convey the message that drinking passengers are safe by focusing exclusively on the boat operators. The epidemiology of boating fatalities suggests that drinking passengers are at risk for falling overboard and that a substantial proportion of boating fatalities occur in this manner. Thus, the current "designated boater" educational effort is incomplete and should be modified to warn about the risks of alcohol use for operators and passengers.[28]

Similarly, a number of popular books on boating instruction either do not mention alcohol in the context of boating, or they simply inform about drinking and boating laws. Even those books that warn about the risks of drinking while operating a boat fail to warn about risks to drinking passengers or risks to individuals who are drinking on boats that are drifting or moored. Writers and publishers of books on boating instruction should be made aware of the need to include or expand sections on drinking and boating.[28]

A recent Red Cross National Boating Survey found that only about one-third of boaters have ever taken a boating course. In addition, the number of boaters who take training courses appears to be declining. In spite of this trend, over one-third of boaters say they would support some form of mandatory boater training.[26]

Even if all boaters were required to participate in some type of training it is not at all clear that training, in its present state, would be sufficient for educating boaters about alcohol and aquatic safety. Current training has not adequately addressed the risks of drinking and boating.[28]

The survey of boaters conducted by the Red Cross also provides evidence that boaters need to receive better information about the risks of drinking and boating. When asked what they would most like to see covered in a training course, the most frequently cited response was information on the causes of, and how to prevent, accidents.[26] This cannot be done thoroughly without explanation of alcohol's role in contributing to drowning and boating mishaps.

More needs to be done to educate boaters about the risks of drinking and boating for both operators and passengers. The National Transportation Safety Board has urged the Educational Committee of the National Association of State Boating Law Administrators to insist that state and national boating safety courses include a comprehensive guide on the risks of using alcohol while boating, as well as the legal and ethical responsibilities of boat captains.[29]

In addition, the Coast Guard should take a more active role in evaluating and defining a model education program, and in disseminating this information to the many other boat training organizations, including the National Safe Boating Council, the National Water Safety Congress, and the Boat Owners Association of the United States.[29]

There are other indications that the current education efforts are inadequate. Only about one-third of the population is even aware that there is a federal law prohibiting the operation of a vessel while intoxicated on federal waterways.[27] In addition, 25% of respondents to a recent national survey had never heard of, or recalled seeing, any information at all on the risks of using alcohol in an aquatic environment.[30]

Research Issues

Risk Factor Studies

Although a case control study on the risk of alcohol for boating fatalities has been conducted[19] and another case control study of the risk of alcohol for nonboating studies is currently underway,[18] these studies alone cannot yield definitive evidence of the causal role of drinking for aquatic injury. Further case control studies will be required to validate the associations determined thus far and to develop better estimates of the magnitude of risks, the levels of blood alcohol at which risk begins to increase, and the dose–response relationship between alcohol exposure and risk.

Case control studies are difficult to execute in aquatic settings. Often there are no witnesses to drownings and therefore it is difficult to know all of the circumstances surrounding the event. This presents problems in terms of identifying suitable controls. Moreover, once identified, aquatic environments can be awkward settings in which to conduct interviews and conduct blood alcohol testing.

Ascertainment of alcohol exposure among victims also presents problems. Reporting of evidence of alcohol following an aquatic death is often not complete and, in many locales, blood alcohol testing of victims is not mandatory and is done at the discretion of local authorities. It is known that the breakdown of tissues submerged for a length of time yields alcohols as a byproduct of decomposition. These alcohols can be difficult to distinguish from ingested alcohols. It is often not known for how long a recovered victim's body has been submerged. However, even if this information was available, our current level of understanding is limited with respect to how rapidly fermentation takes place or of the relationship between, say, fermentation and water temperature.

Physiological Effects of Alcohol

Alcohol can contribute to aquatic injury via several pathways. First, alcohol can increase the likelihood of a precipitating event such as falling off a boat. Next, alcohol can impair the ability to respond effectively to a life-threatening event, regardless of whether that event was initially caused by drinking. Third, even small amounts of alcohol may compromise physiological systems in ways that increase risk for drowning.

Although there are many hypotheses about how alcohol might interact with aquatic exposures to produce physiological responses potentiating drowning, there have been few studies performed to test these hypotheses. More research is needed on the effects of the interaction between exposure to water and alcohol on cardiac response, balance and orientation, body temperature, and blood-gas sensing.

The risks of drinking for boat passengers, as opposed to boat operators, needs further clarification. As noted earlier, boating differs from vehicular driving in that drunken passengers in cars are relatively safe as long as the car operators are sober. This is probably not the case with boat passengers, who are at risk of falling overboard even if the boat operator has not been drinking. More detailed case studies of boating fatalities are required to sort out the respective role of operators vs passengers in precipitating fatal boating events.

Discussion

There are several reasons why drinking in aquatic settings should be of concern to public health policymakers and practitioners. First, although further research is needed on the causal role of alcohol in aquatic injury and deaths, evidence to date suggests that drinking substantially increases the risk for drowning. Second, our national survey indicates that a very large proportion of the population has at least some degree of exposure to aquatic settings. Third, our survey also indicates that drinking commonly accompanies aquatic activities. Although the number of drownings is relatively small, and decreasing over time, the risks of drinking in aquatic settings may be as great, or higher, than the risks posed by drinking and driving. At present, there are about 10 times as many vehicular deaths as drownings (which make up the large majority of aquatic deaths). It is very likely, however, that on average individuals spend many more hours in automobiles than on or near the water. Thus, per unit of exposure, drowning rates probably exceed vehicular death rates and alcohol-related drowning rates may exceed drunken driving fatality rates when calculated controlling for exposure to vehicles and aquatic settings.

Finally, alcohol-related aquatic deaths could probably be reduced without extensive use of additional public health resources. The extent of drinking in aquatic settings suggests that the public considers this behavior normative. These attitudes are reinforced by commercial advertisements depicting alcohol use in aquatic settings and by public information campaigns that focus on drinking boat operators but fail to warn boat passengers about the risks of alcohol. More extensive and accurate information campaigns about the risks of drinking in aquatic settings could, at a minimum, inform the public and ultimately affect norms about drinking on or near the water.

References

[1]National Safety Council (1992) *Accident Facts 1992 Edition.* Author, Itasca, IL.

[2]US Coast Guard. *Boating Statistics 1991.* Commandant Publication P16754.1., June 1992, US Coast Guard, Washington, DC.

[3]C. Branche-Dorsey, S. M. Smith, and D. Johnson, Centers for Disease Control and Prevention (1993) *A study of boat and boat propeller-related injury in the United States: 1991–1992.* Presented at the Second World Conference on Injury Control, March 1993, Atlanta, GA.

[4]J. Howland and R. Hingson (1988) Alcohol as a risk factor for drowning: a review of the literature (1950–1985). *Accident Anal. Prev.* **20,** 19–25.

[5]R. Hingson and J. Howland (1993) Alcohol and non-traffic unintended injuries. *Addiction* **88,** 877–883.

[6]G. S. Smith and J. F. Kraus (1988) Alcohol and residential, recreational, and occupational injuries: a review of the epidemiologic evidence. *Annu. Rev. Public Health* **9,** 99–121.

[7]V. D. Plueckhahn (1984) Alcohol and accidental drowning: a 25-year study. *Med. J. Australia* **141(1),** 22–25.

[8]J. A. Waller (1972) Nonhighway injury fatalities-I. The role of alcohol and problem drinking, drugs, and medical impairment. *J. Chron. Dis.* **25,** 33–45.

[9]P. Deitz and S. Baker (1974) Drowning epidemiology and prevention. *Am. J. Public Health* **64,** 303–312.

[10]R. Berkelman, J. Herndon, J. Callaway, R. Stevens, L. Howard, A. Bezjak, and R. Sikes (1990) Fatal injuries and alcohol. *Am. J. Prev. Med.* **1,** 21–28.

[11]G. Wintemute, J. Kraus, S. Teret, and M. Wright (1988) The epidemiology of drowning in adulthood: implications for prevention. *Am. J. Prev. Med.* **4,** 343–348.

[12]A. Altwicker and J. Howland (1990) *Alcohol and recreational boating fatalities.* Presented at the 118th American Public Health Association Annual Meeting, New York.

[13]W. R. Katkin, W. N. Hayes, A. I. Tegor, and D. G. Pruitt (1970) Effects of alcoholic beverages differing in congener content on psychomotor tasks and risk taking. *Q. J. Stud. Alcohol* **31(Suppl. 5),** 105–114.

[14]M. W. Perrine (1973) Alcohol's influences on driving-related behavior: a critical review of laboratory studies of neurophysiological, neuromuscular, and sensory activity. *J. Safety Res.* **5,** 165–184

[15]National Transportation Safety Board (1983) *Recreational Boating Safety and Alcohol.* NTSB/55-83/02, Washington, DC.

[16]B. Gooden (1984) Drowning and alcohol. *Med. J. Australia* **141,** 478.

[17]C. Stiehl (1975) *Alcohol and Pleasure Boat Operators.* United States Coast Guard, Report CGD13475, Washington, DC.

[18]G. S. Smith (1993) *Alcohol and Drowning Risk: Preliminary Report on Drowning Study.* Unpublished report, Johns Hopkins School of Hygiene and Public Health, Baltimore, MD.

[19]P. Mengert, E. D. Sussman, and R. DiSario (1992) *A Study of the Relationship Between the Risk of Fatality and Blood Alcohol Concentration of Recreational Boat Operators.* Report CG-D-09-92, US Coast Guard, Washington, DC.

[20]J. Howland et al. (1994) *Alcohol Use in Aquatic Settings: Results of a National Survey.* Unpublished report.

²¹A. Penttila, S. Piipponen, and J. Pikkarinen (1979) Drunken driving with motorboats in Finland. *Accident Anal. Prev.* **11,** 237–239.

²²US Coast Guard, US Department of Transportation (1978) *Recreational Boating in the U.S. in 1973 and 1976: The Nationwide Boating Survey.* Report No. CG-13-003-75, Washington, DC.

²³Boat/US Foundation for Boating Safety (1984) *Alcohol and Boating Survey.* Alexandria, VA.

²⁴E. D. Glover and S. M. Lane (1989) *Prevalence of Alcohol Consumption and Recreational Boating in Beaufort County, North Carolina.* American Public Health Association 117th Annual Meeting, Chicago, October 22–26.

²⁵J. Howland, T. Mangione, R. Hingson, M. Levenson, and A. Altwicker (1990) A pilot survey of aquatic activities and related consumption of alcohol with implications for drowning. *Public Health Rep.* **105,** 415–419.

²⁶The American Red Cross (1991) *American Red Cross National Boating Survey.* Washington, DC.

²⁷J. Howland (1992) *Drinking and Boating—Results of a National Survey.* The Secretary's Conference on Alcohol-Related Injuries, Washington, DC.

²⁸J. Howland, G. S. Smith, T. Mangione, R. Hingson, W. DeJong, and N. Bell (1993) Missing the boat on drinking and boating. *JAMA* **270,** 91,92.

²⁹National Transportation Safety Board (1993) *Safety Study—Recreational Boating Safety and Alcohol.* National Transportation Safety Board, Bureau of Safety Programs, October 17, Washington, DC.

³⁰J. Howland, R. Hingson, T. Heeren, S. Bak, and T. Mangione (1993) Alcohol use and aquatic activities, United States, 1991. *Morbid. Mortal. Wkly. Rep.* **42(35),** 675–682.

The Role of Treatment in Reducing Alcohol-Related Accidents Involving DWI Offenders

William F. Wieczorek

Introduction

The problems posed to the safety of the general public by alcohol-impaired drivers are well known and constitute a substantial public health risk.[1,2] Alcohol is implicated in about 5% of property damage traffic accidents and about 10% of personal injury accidents each year.[3-5] Depending on the estimate of the total number of traffic accidents in a year (accidents known to police vs estimates of total accidents), alcohol is involved in 180,000–1.2 million property crashes and 200,000–300,000 personal injury crashes.[3,5] Although alcohol-related traffic fatalities have decreased somewhat during the 1980s, they continue to account for 40–50% of the fatal crashes.[6] Despite efforts in a number of areas, such as increased enforcement, raising the legal drinking age, legislation to increase penalties for driving while intoxicated (DWI), and increased public awareness campaigns (e.g., Mothers Against Drunk Driving, Students Against Drunk Driving, Remove Intoxicated Drivers), alcohol-related accidents and their associated costs in dollars and lives will continue as major public health and traffic safety problem for the foreseeable future. Thus, there is an ongoing need for programs and approaches that could be effective in reducing any or all parts of this alcohol/traffic accident problem.

From: *Drug and Alcohol Abuse Reviews, Vol. 7: Alcohol, Cocaine, and Accidents*
Ed.: R. R. Watson ©1995 Humana Press Inc., Totowa, NJ

This chapter provides a critical examination of the role of treatment for DWI offenders in reducing alcohol-related accidents. The purpose is to focus on recent developments and major issues pertaining to treatment approaches for DWI offenders, not to provide an exhaustive review of the literature. Some definitions are needed before moving on to more substantive issues. The term "DWI offenders" is used in this chapter to describe persons who were convicted of any drinking and driving offense. "Treatment" is the term used to describe an intervention designed to eliminate or reduce drinking and associated problems such as impaired driving and other risky behaviors. A "treatment intervention" may consist of any combination of education, counseling, and other therapy such as pharmacotherapy.

Also, "accidents" will be the term used to describe incidents that involve personal and/or property damage resulting from the operation of a motor vehicle, although the term "crash" will also be used as a synonym to avoid over-repetition. The intent of the participants is of major interest because individuals may choose to elevate the probability of an accident by participating in risk-enhancing behaviors (e.g., speeding, drinking, and drug use). However, almost no one engages in higher risk behaviors with the intention of being in or causing an accident.

The linkage between drinking and accidents is rather tenuous to an individual driver. The absolute probability of any accident for an alcohol impaired driver is very low (considerably less than 1%),[7] although the risk increases as blood alcohol content rises. A driver with a blood alcohol content of about .15% has an approx 350-fold increase in the risk of a single-vehicle fatal accident compared to a nondrinking driver.[1] The driver has the main role in avoiding or causing accidents; however, it is important to be cognizant of the complex multifactorial genesis of accidents. Drivers are an appropriate focus for safety efforts, but not to the exclusion of other human and nonhuman factors.[8,9] The problem is that the trend toward using crashes distorts the assessment of accidents toward sole blame on the driver. Culpability should be assessed individually for each case and include an assessment of the drivers' actual blood alcohol content, risky driving behaviors, and context of the behavior.[10]

DWI Offenders as a Target for Treatment

Multiple approaches are necessary to reduce the number of alcohol-impaired drivers and accidents. The Surgeon General's Workshop on Drunk Driving[11] and Ross's recent book[10] provide excellent overviews of a number of policies to reduce DWI. These policy options include transportation alternatives, highway improvements, criminal justice approaches, vehicle design changes, advertising regulations, alcohol control efforts, primary prevention/education, and treatment programs.

DWI offenders are an important target population for treatment efforts in the United States. DWI is the largest single offense for arrests in the United States. About 1.8 million DWI arrests were made in 1990.[12] More than 1 million persons are convicted of DWI each year, producing a large pool of persons officially identified as misusing alcohol. The review by Vingilis[13] concluded that a reasonable estimate of the proportion of DWI offenders who could be considered to be alcoholics or alcohol dependent is about 50%, depending on the definition of alcoholism that is used. Thus, many of these individuals have alcohol problems that could benefit from organized treatment.

Miller and Windle[14] more recently reviewed issues concerning the measurement of problem drinking among DWI offenders and suggested the need for better instruments and assessment in this area. Using criteria based on *DSM–III–R*,[15] Wieczorek and colleagues[16] found that 51% of a sample of DWI offenders referred for alcoholism evaluation were alcohol dependent. Further research used *DSM–III–R* alcohol diagnosis based on a modified version of the Diagnostic Interview Schedule (DIS)[17] in a sample of first and repeat DWI offenders. Diagnosis was common as 62% of DWI first offenders and 84% of repeat offenders were alcohol dependent.[18] Thus, ample evidence clearly indicates that a substantial proportion of DWI offenders are in need of treatment for their alcohol problems. The DWI arrest statistics and research on alcohol dependence among DWI offenders suggests that about 500,000 DWI offenders each year may need treatment.

Is There a Role
for Treatment in Reducing Accidents?

Treatment for DWI offenders can be strongly justified in terms of the possible improvement in the offenders' health and social functioning. Significant public health objectives pertaining to family function, occupational stability, and physical health are associated with decreased alcohol consumption by problem drinkers such as most DWI offenders. However, the issue of whether treatment can have an impact on alcohol-related traffic accidents deserves greater attention.

The prevailing wisdom on this matter, presented by Stewart and Ellingstad,[19] is that "rehabilitative approaches can only have a very small effect on traffic safety, even if maximally effective" (p. 243). Recent research findings cast doubt on this conventional wisdom. A substantial number of alcohol-related fatal accidents may be avoided through effective treatment programs if DWI offenders are a sizable proportion of the drivers in alcohol-related fatalities. Information indicating that treatment could have a meaningful effect on accidents would be a sufficient reason for re-evaluating the role of treatment in reducing accidents.

Fell recently reported on the proportion of drivers involved in fatal collisions who had a DWI conviction in the 3 yr prior to the fatality.[20] Using data from the Fatal Accident Reporting System (FARS), this research found that about 10% of the drivers in alcohol-related fatalities had a DWI conviction in the previous 3 yr. Almost 12% of the drivers with blood alcohol concentrations (BACs) over .10 and about 6% of the drivers with BACs of .01–.09 had a previous DWI conviction. An even higher rate was found in New Zealand where over 25% of the drivers in fatal collisions had a previous DWI conviction.[21]

The proportion of drivers in alcohol-related fatalities with previous DWI convictions is likely to be higher than 10%. Fell recommended that the estimates he presented should be preceded by the phrase "at the minimum" because of limitations in the data.[20] The information on the fatal crash was based on a limited time frame (3 yr), did not cover DWIs received in a state other than where the crash was located, and did not take into account DWI arrests that did not lead to a conviction. All of these factors suggest that the potential impact for treatment on alcohol-related traffic fatalities may substantially exceed 10%. Therefore, the maximum impact of treatment on alcohol-related traffic fatalities is much more than Reed's[22] estimate of about 2.5%. Furthermore, the lower rate of impaired driving found by Lund and Wolf,[23] coupled with a steady number of DWI arrests, would increase the potential savings that could be provided by effective treatment because a greater proportion of the total drinking-driving population is included in the DWI arrestee population. So as enforcement and primary prevention become more effective, the potential impact of treatment will increase.

Even if treatment is not 100% effective, and we certainly have ample evidence of this, the potential gain in lives saved by treatment is meaningful. If treatment were effective in reducing only 50% of the alcohol-related traffic fatalities associated with known DWI offenders, it would amount to about 1000 lives saved each year. This estimate is based on the FARS data presented by Fell which showed that a total of 1965 drivers in fatal crashes involving alcohol were previous DWI offenders. These findings provide strong evidence that effective treatment could be a part of an integrated approach to minimizing alcohol-related accidents. In addition, the reduction in alcohol-related accidents that could result from treatment are comparable to that which could be expected from other interventions such as road blocks, server intervention, and drinking age laws.[10,24]

DWI treatment can be further justified on a cost/benefit basis even if the potential impact on total alcohol-related fatalities did not exist. In addition, treatment for DWI is not a burden to the current system of arrest and adjudication because the cost of treatment is usually met by the DWI offender. If treatment for DWI offenders results in improved health and general functioning that leads to decreased accident-related mortality, then the benefit of treatment greatly exceeds the costs to both the individual and society, regardless of who paid for the treatment.

Brief Review
of DWI Treatment Outcomes

This section presents a brief overview of DWI treatment outcomes to provide an introduction to:

1. The types of treatment experienced by DWI offenders;
2. The level of success associated with treatment for DWI offenders;
3. Some of the problems associated with this research; and
4. Update the more complete reviews of this literature.

Comprehensive reviews of DWI treatment programs are provided by Foon,[25] Mann et al.,[26] and Stewart and Ellingstad.[18] In addition, rearrest for DWI is the outcome measure most commonly used to evaluate treatment for DWI offenders. Motor vehicle accidents, especially those not related to drinking, are not commonly used to evaluate treatment, although when they are the results are similar to those found for recidivism.[26]

DWI offenders are exposed to a wide variety of treatments. Educational programs modeled after the Phoenix program of the early 1970s[27] are common. These educational programs may vary somewhat in content but usually emphasize facts pertaining to alcohol, the consequences of impaired driving, and ways to avoid drinking and driving. Therapy programs tailored specifically for DWI offenders are uncommon, although there are some exceptions (e.g., Siegal,[28] Voas and Tippetts,[29] and Washousky[30]). DWI offenders participate in all types of therapy including in-patient programs, individualized outpatient counseling, pharmacotherapy, group and behavioral programs, self-help programs (e.g., Alcoholics Anonymous [AA]), and others.[31]

A major problem in assessing the impact of education and treatment programs for DWI offenders is the lack of methodological rigor in many studies.[25,26,32,33] These difficulties include:

1. Problems with research strategies such as inadequate control groups;
2. Inadequate outcome measures; and
3. Questionable assessment procedures including problems with the validity of problem drinker assessments.

Note that most outcome studies of DWI offenders do not examine accidents as an outcome measure. There are several reasons for this. The official data available on accidents are often incomplete, many property damage collisions are never reported, and alcohol involvement is assessed inconsistently.

The Alcohol Safety Action Programs (ASAP), developed nationally in the early 1970s, provided the stimulus for DWI interventions consisting of educational programs coupled with referral to alcoholism rehabilitation.[34] Nichols and associates[35] reviewed the impact of the ASAPs, finding that methodologically poor evaluations (e.g., lack of control group or no differentiation of drinker types by outcome) tended to find more positive outcomes for both the educational and treatment modalities than did more methodologically sound studies.

One methodologically sound evaluation of 11 ASAPs assessed educational and treatment modalities using random assignment and an 18-mo followup.[36,37] The only notable difference between treatment and control groups in either modality was a lower rearrest rate for the education group in mo 15–18. This result, however, may be owing to positive outcomes at ASAP sites that used small-group interaction programs that may be more like rehabilitation than education.[26] A common finding in the literature is that knowledge and attitudes toward drinking and driving are often improved after an educational program, whereas drinking outcomes are not.[38–41]

More recent research evaluated educational and treatment programs while taking offender and treatment type into consideration. Mixed results characterize the findings pertaining to low alcohol problem offenders, defined by first offender status or a measure of alcohol problems, in educational programs. In well-designed studies of first offenders, Blount et al.[42] and Essex and Weinerth[43] reported less recidivism for program participants, whereas Holden[44] and Landrum et al.[45] reported no impact for an educational program on low-alcohol problem individuals.

Landrum et al.[45] noted a marginal impact for education plus probation for low problem offenders, which was not replicated in a longer term followup of the same sample.[46] Reis[47] randomly assigned DWI first offenders to a four-session education program, a take-home study course, or a no-treatment control group, finding no significant difference between groups after about 2 yr. After an additional 18 mo, however, both education groups showed less recidivism than the controls.[48] Evaluations of the impact of educational programs on repeat offenders or problem drinkers have found no evidence for the efficacy of these programs for higher problem DWI offenders.[41,44,45]

Evaluations have even found negative impacts for some treatment programs. McGuire[49] found significantly worse outcomes for heavy drinkers treated by such modalities as AA and individual therapy when compared with untreated heavy drinkers. Nichols et al.[50] found a negative impact for Power Motivation Training on the treatment group when compared to the control group receiving no treatment. Reis[48] examined recidivism rates of multiple DWI offenders who received either eclectic group counseling for 1 yr (some individuals also received disulfiram but showed no difference in outcome from the others in this group), brief individual contacts (15 min) every other week for 1 yr, or a no-treatment control group. Over approx 3 yr, those in counseling had a significantly lower recidivism rate than the controls. In contrast, Holden[44] found no impact on DWI rearrest rates for treatment, education, or supervision of individuals classified as problem drinkers when compared to a control group.

The Weekend Intervention Program (WIP) was developed by Siegal[28,51] as an intense assessment and initial therapy for DWI offenders. In a naturalistic study (the courts would not support random assignment) of 3556 DWI offenders, Siegal found marginally significant reductions ($p = .05$) in DWI recidivism for repeat offenders who were mandated to comply with the WIP treatment recommendations. The reduction in recidivism was not statistically significant for the first offenders.

Voas and Tippetts[29] evaluated the impact of a residential 28-d facility for DWI offenders and a long-term monitoring program that included treatment for alcohol problems. The main result was a significant reduction in overall recidivism for those who participated in either (or both) the facility and monitoring programs. This effect was largest in the first year when the control group had four times more recidivism. However, data limitations made it impossible to know whether these results were most applicable to first or repeat offenders.

A comparison of a coping skills intervention, a single contact drinking-driving session, and a control group performed by Donovan and associates[52] using DWI first offenders found some encouraging results. The coping skills group showed the greatest decrease in alcohol consumption and both the control group and the coping skills group had fewer moving violations than the single-contact group. However, DWI recidivism did not differ significantly because of sample size limitations, although the trend was toward a lower rate in the coping skills group.

Nochajski et al.[53] examined the impact of a Drinking Driver Evaluation and Treatment designed for severe DWI offenders referred by the courts and/or the Department of Motor Vehicles. The results showed a differential impact based on criminal history; those with arrests for crimes other than DWI were more than twice as likely to be rearrested for DWI.

Mann and colleagues[54] examined the mortality of treated vs untreated repeat DWI offenders. A long-term followup of the mortality among these DWI offenders found that the treatment group had significantly less mortality than expected. The largest difference in mortality between the groups was due to the treated group having only about 25% of the expected mortality from accidental and violent death.

At best, the literature on DWI treatment provides limited support for positive outcomes. There is some evidence that suggests differential outcomes based on offender characteristics (first vs repeat, problem vs nonproblem drinker) and for different types programs (education vs therapy).

Developments that Could Improve DWI Treatment Outcomes

The limitations found for DWI treatment should not be discouraging because the findings pertaining to differential outcomes for specific groups indicate that positive treatment impact is possible. Also, research suggests that DWI offenders select the least intrusive treatment program acceptable for relicensing requirements rather than the most clinically appropriate treatment.[31] Therefore, efforts to match certain types of DWI offenders to the most appropriate treatment are needed. This idea of matching treatment to the offender, which is often called treatment matching, has been in the DWI literature for some time. However, the treatment matching found in the literature for DWI offenders is rudimentary because all high problem subjects are matched with higher intensity treatments. Thus, many DWI outcome studies are reports on outcomes for specific modalities rather than examinations of the efficacy of treatment matching, which requires mismatched cases for an adequate evaluation.

A number of researchers in the DWI field have recognized the potential of treatment matching for improving DWI outcomes.[55–58] Mann[56] recently pointed out the matching possibilities for DWI offenders that are suggested by the differential outcomes based on problem severity found in the ASAP studies. Wells-Parker and coworkers[57] also reviewed findings, particularly in the area of demographic variables, that suggest a role for treatment matching for DWI offenders. Treatment matching should be viewed as part of a developing program of research on DWI treatment. Researchers in this area have identified alcoholism treatment matching as an area that can provide substantial guidance to DWI treatment matching efforts because the large overlap in DWI and alcoholic populations provides great commonality and the research on alcoholism treatment matching is at a more mature level of development.[58,59]

Alcoholism Treatment Matching

One way to increase the efficiency and effectiveness of DWI-offender treatment is to appropriately match offender characteristics to the type and style of the treatment, a concept known as the treatment-matching hypothesis. The matching hypothesis was suggested some time ago,[60] and recently has become a focus for alcoholism treatment research.[61–63] The utility of borrowing from the alcoholism-matching literature for the development of matching approaches for DWI offenders has been clearly recognized by Donovan and Rosengren,[59] who also provided a detailed overview of alcoholism treatment-matching issues.

Matching criteria found to result in differential outcomes for alcoholics form four groups (*see* Committee to Identify Research Opportunities in the Prevention and Treatment of Alcohol-Related Problems,[64] Donovan and Rosengren,[59] Miller,[63] and Miller and Hester[65] for reviews).

Severity of Alcohol Dependence

Alcoholics characterized by loss of control drinking and physical dependence had more positive outcomes when they received intensive treatment vs a brief intervention, whereas problem drinkers (no physical dependence) fared better after the brief intervention than after intensive treatment.[66] Two groups of alcoholics (high- and low-severity alcohol dependence) were randomly matched with a higher intensity, structured, coping skills group, or a lower intensity, interactional-focus group.[67] The high-dependency group did better in the more structured atmosphere than they did in the interaction groups. The opposite was true for low dependence alcoholics.

Psychiatric Problems

Poorer treatment outcomes for alcohol dependence are associated with a global measure of psychopathology and with specific diagnoses for men and women.[68] McLellan and associates[69] performed treatment matching based on the psychiatric severity of alcoholics. The number, duration, and intensity of psychiatric symptomatology on intake was operationalized into low, medium, and high categories. High severity alcoholics were excluded from the analysis because a previous study found that this group responded negatively to the modalities available.[70] The findings for the low and medium psychiatric severity groups (e.g., the lower severity group did better in lower impact treatment) supported the use of treatment matching. Kadden et al.[71] randomly assigned alcoholic in-patients to either coping skills training or interactional therapy. Subjects higher in sociopathy and psychopathology had better outcomes after social skills training. Lower sociopathy individuals did better after the interactional therapy.

Personality

An early matching study used the personality construct called conceptual level for matching alcoholics to therapists.[72] Patients matched with a therapist of similar conceptual level had much more positive outcomes than those who were mismatched.[72] Similar results were found for matching during treatment aftercare.[73] Annis and Chan[74] performed a random assignment of alcohol and drug abusing criminal offenders to intensive, 8-wk group therapy, or to routine institutional care. The assignments were based on an empirically derived personality factor called self-image, based mainly on self-esteem and control orientation. Offenders receiving group therapy who were high in self-image had more positive outcomes than the institutional group. Persons low in self-image and treated with group therapy actually had more negative outcomes than the institutional control group.

Social Stability

Social stability (e.g., being employed, married, and of higher socio-economic status) has long been associated with positive alcoholism treatment outcomes.[64,75] The importance of general social support is shown by the finding that community reinforcement enhanced treatment outcomes for unmarried alcoholics, but not for married ones.[76]

In addition, some recent research findings are particularly supportive of approaches available and previously used in the DWI field. A comprehensive review of alcohol typologies concluded that empirical clustering techniques may be the most appropriate approach to finding meaningful subtypes.[77] More importantly, Babor et al.[78] empirically derived a cluster-based typology of alcoholics. This typology had two groups: one group, called type A, was less severely dependent and had less risk factors and symptoms, whereas the other group, called type B, had greater dependence severity (despite younger age) and more risk factors and problems. A treatment-matching and outcome study of 79 alcoholics showed that the type A group had better outcomes after coping skills treatment, whereas the type B group had better outcomes after interactional therapy.[79]

DWI Heterogeneity and Matching

Research has clearly shown that DWI offenders are a population characterized by a significant amount of heterogeneity.[2,14,80,81] The recognition of DWI heterogeneity has led to a focus on identifying subgroups based on either a single distinguishing characteristic or on multiple variables. A variety of domains that could be relevant to treatment matching have been recognized in the literature. The fact that alcohol diagnoses and the severity of problem drinking varies among DWI offenders has been recognized for quite some time.[13,14] DWI offenders are differentiated by their levels of psychological problems[14] and psychiatric symptomatology.[82] Personality measures such as sensation seeking, risk taking, and aggression are known to identify subgroups of DWI offenders.[83,84] Demographic characteristics such as age and social stability may also be useful for matching.[57,59]

Two notable domains that could have clinical relevance are criminal history and high-risk driving. Criminal history for offenses other than drinking and driving are relatively common among DWI offenders[85,86] and has been predictive of DWI recidivism.[53] Criminal history may provide a method to characterize the severity of sociopathy among DWI offenders. Research by MacDonald[87,88] suggested that alcoholics who are DWI offenders and have a history of motor vehicle accidents tend to display characteristics associated with antisocial personalities. High-risk driving is an especially appropriate area to focus efforts to reduce accidents among DWI offenders. Donovan and coworkers[89] concluded that DWI offenders are a subgroup of the larger high-risk driving population. High-risk drivers, as identified by their moving violations, were found to become DWI offenders at a rate five times greater than for the general driver population.[90] There is likely to be some overlap between antisocial personality and high-risk drivers because aggressive and impulsive behaviors characterize both groups.

These subgroupings of DWI offenders should have clinical utility for DWI treatment matching. However, there is no research that follows through on the promise of using subgroup characteristics to identify and develop effective treatments or interventions. In addition, multivariate classifications or typologies may be more fruitful because multiple domains are incorporated.

DWI Typologies and Treatment Matching

Multivariate typologies show strong potential for identifying relevant treatment-related characteristics in the DWI population.[58,91–96] Three multivariate typologies (Donovan and Marlatt,[92] Steer et al.,[94] and Wieczorek and Miller[58]) are noteworthy for their DWI treatment implications.

Steer et al.[94] used a cluster procedure to recognize seven groups of DWI offenders based on BAC at arrest, alcohol quantity frequency, an alcohol impairment index, and a psychoneuroticism stability scale. About 37% of the sample fell into a low alcohol/psychological impairment group, a common finding in this area. Some groups, such as a self-medicating group and a high alcohol and psychological problem group, had characteristics that could be matched with specific modalities; however, no treatment matching was done.

Donovan and Marlatt[92] identified five clusters based on personality (e.g., sensation seeking, control orientation, and hostility), two of which were considered high risks for continued drinking and driving. One high-risk cluster was characterized by an elevated level of tension-reduction driving and low levels of depression and resentment. High levels of driving-related aggression, competitive speed, sensation seeking, and hostility typified the other high-risk cluster. Three-year followup data showed the two high-risk groups to have significantly more nonalcohol traffic violations than the other clusters, but no differences on alcohol-related crashes and violations.[97] This study showed:

1. The need for interventions to improve the driving skills of DWI offenders;
2. That typologies of DWI offenders could have predictive validity; and
3. That future typologies should include direct measures of alcohol use/ problems.

A preliminary typology has been developed that clearly shows the advantages of a theory-based classification for treatment-matching purposes.[58] Wieczorek and Miller[58] used cluster analysis to develop the only DWI typology specifically designed to facilitate treatment matching. The typology was derived from four variables (severity of alcohol dependence, psychiatric severity, social instability, and bad-driving index) selected to facilitate treatment-matching decisions pertaining to the areas in need of treatment (alcohol, driving, or both), the intensity of the treatment, and the focus of the treatment (problem focused vs broad spectrum). Two cluster procedures and external validation were used to derive a total of five clusters. Similar to other DWI typologies, the largest cluster (31% of the cases) was a low-problem severity group.[92,96] The typology also included a high-risk driver group (5% of the cases), a moderate severity cluster (26%), a socially stable high-problem severity cluster (15%), and a socially instable high-problem severity cluster (24%).

At this stage of development, treatment recommendations suitable for the groups in this typology are treatment-matching hypotheses that need to be examined by research before implementation can be considered. However, the process of examining DWI subgroups and matching their characteristics to an intervention plan can illustrate the utility of the approach. The low-problem cluster would appear to be best served by participation in drinking and driving education courses. The moderate severity group would appear to require a low-intensity alcohol treatment and a program to enhance driving skills. The high-risk driver group showed a need for both drinking and driving treatments with the alcohol component at a moderate intensity and the most intensive driving component available. The socially instable high-severity group requires the most intensive overall package of treatment. A broad spectrum in-patient program with aftercare components that focus on improving social stability are warranted. A high-intensity broad spectrum program would seem most appropriate for the socially stable high-severity group. Much work remains to be done before the promise of treatment matching can be realized. Important questions regarding which type of treatment is most appropriate for specific subgroups are currently unanswered because the treatment-matching field is still in an early stage of development.

The typology clearly shows the feasibility of the methodology and strongly suggests some specific matching hypotheses pertaining to the type of treatment most appropriate for each group. This typology is designed to support treatment matching at the initial stage where the type of treatment (alcohol, psychiatric, or driving), intensity of the treatment, and the treatment focus is selected. More detailed matching may be appropriate at the level of interaction between the client and a clinician. However, this typology begins to provide a methodology for providing the criminal justice system and motor vehicle agencies with guidance to the type of treatment that would be most appropriate for DWI offenders.

A recent examination of cluster-based classifications of DWI offenders raised some issues concerning their utility. Wells-Parker et al.[98] found it difficult to replicate their cluster results, and suggested that utilizing underlying dimensions may be more appropriate than typologies. The analyses in this article, however, used a large number of variables (about 40) for the cluster derivations. The variance of such a large number of measures will tend to be randomly spread over hyperspace, which obscures the clusters. This problem of too many and/or irrelevant variables producing "noisy" data has been recognized in the cluster analytic literature.[99,100] In addition, the researchers relied on a single coefficient to define the existence of "true" clusters, whereas a convergent approach using several indicators of the number of clusters would be better advised.[100] Moreover, the recent findings cited in the earlier section on Alcoholism Treatment Matching showed that multivariate typologies for alcoholics were useful for treatment matching and had predictive value for treatment outcomes. However, this should not discourage future efforts to examine dimensions or factors for facilitating treatment matching for DWI offenders.

Although DWI research pertaining to subgroups and distinguishing characteristics alludes to the need for treatment matching with DWI populations, almost no research has attempted it. When attempts to match are found in the DWI literature,[46] all high-problem individuals are given more intensive treatment than the low-problem individuals. This procedure does not allow for a proper assessment since there are no mismatched cases. There also is a failure to match on domains other than the severity of alcohol problems, although the DWI subgroup literature identifies salient problem areas such as criminal history[85] and personality.[101] Additional matching criteria are suggested in the treatment-matching literature on alcoholism.

Treatment vs Sanctions

The purpose of treatment and treatment matching for DWI offenders is to improve the probability of positive outcomes, including a reduction in accidents, not to divert offenders away from appropriate legal sanctions. A substantial body of literature indicates that sanctions for DWI, such as license suspension, provide a more effective improvement in traffic safety when compared with treatment, particularly when treatment is used as a substitute for a sanction.[24,102,103] This does not mean that treatment should be abandoned, but that treatment in lieu of sanctions is not effective.

Treatment can also be thought of as an additional sanction. The cost of treatment is usually paid by the DWI offender either directly or through a third party, such as a health insurance company. When treatment costs are paid directly by the offender, the costs are similar to an increased fine for the DWI offense. Treatment also places constraints on the behavior of the DWI offender, which are similar to prohibitions included in sanctions such as reduced or no alcohol consumption. However, only when treatment is mandated by either the courts or a motor vehicle licensing agency is it truly a sanction. Allowing the offender to select treatment instead of another punishment decreases and may even nullify the impact of treatment as a sanction.

Table 1
Key Components of Treatment Matching for DWI Offenders

Theory-based matching concepts
Adequate assessment for matching assignment and control variables
Appropriate treatment program for matched cases
Include mismatched cases (e.g., random assignment or quasi-
    experimental design)
Adequate outcome measures
Sufficient followups (both in number and time after the treatment)

Treatment and sanctions should be seen as complementary approaches to the reduction of alcohol-related accidents. Unfortunately, treatment has been viewed as an alternative and not an adjunct to punishment and the research literature lacks studies that examine the combined effects.

Future Directions

The previous sections of this chapter provided a broad overview of the role of treatment in reducing accidents among DWI offenders. One major point is that the discussion has often focused on the potential reduction in accidents that could be achieved through appropriate DWI treatment. A substantial amount of research is needed for the development of an information base that could be used by policymakers to implement more effective treatments for DWI. The following are the main topics that need to be addressed and include recommendations appropriate for research and some that are directed at policymakers.

Treatment-Matching Research
Is Needed that Focuses on DWI Offenders

The findings on DWI subgroup characteristics and the alcoholism research on treatment matching provide valuable information for designing research on DWI treatment matching. Research is needed in all areas of matching including the examination of single variables for matching (e.g., criminal history)[53,85] and more sophisticated studies using multivariate classifications (e.g., Wieczorek and Miller).[58] For treatment matching to become commonplace for DWI offenders, research must show that a system for assessment and treatment assignment is feasible. Table 1 shows the key components for performing treatment-matching research for DWI offenders. Substantial effort will be needed to successfully accomplish each of the components in any DWI research project. Most of the issues are discussed in this chapter and Mann and Vingilis[104] and Donovan[105] discuss assessment issues.

Current DWI Treatments Need to Be Examined and New Treatments Developed

The DWI subgroup and typology literature provides ideas on the type of problems that treatment needs to address (e.g., alcohol dependence, risk taking, psychiatric problems, poor driving skills). However, before new treatments are developed, available treatments require closer scrutiny. The impact of driver improvement courses should be evaluated to determine whether new treatment modalities are necessary in this specific area relating to traffic safety and accidents.

DWI Outcomes (e.g., Recidivism, Accidents) Need to Be Examined Separately for DWI Subgroups

Much information valuable to the design of treatment matching efforts for DWI offenders could be gained by a systematic evaluation of DWI outcomes by subgroups. The limited amount of data in this area strongly indicate that differential outcomes for DWI subgroups are common. Significant treatment effects for specific subgroups can be missed when all the cases are combined because the average effect masks the positive outcomes that may exist for a specific subgroup. Even in DWI outcome evaluations based on official records, it may be possible to examine outcomes by subgroups defined by such variables as age, sex, driving record, and criminal history. Ideas for matching possibilities and new treatments could result from these efforts. Finally, adequate measures of confounding variables such as previous treatment history, demographics, and driving exposure are necessary to avoid spurious results.

Treatment and Sanctions Need to Be Combined Both in Practice and in DWI Outcome Evaluations

Research has provided compelling evidence that treatment should not be substituted for sanctions in the DWI population. However, research that examines the combined effects of treatment and sanctions is lacking. This research is important because the combined effect of treatment and sanctions may exceed the impact of either separately. The possibility that certain sanctions may increase the efficacy of some treatments is information vital to the development of comprehensive DWI matching programs.

Improved Measures of DWI Outcomes Are Needed

The traffic safety measures typically used to evaluate DWI outcomes (e.g., recidivism, officially recorded accidents, and traffic law violations) provide an inadequate database. These official measures tend to record rare events which are affected by a wide variety of factors such as changes in enforcement practices and on-the-scene evaluations of whether alcohol was involved in a nonfatal accident. Significant variance between jurisdictions and changes over time within a jurisdiction impact on these measures. Accidents that are not the fault of the DWI offender cannot usually be determined from official records, which further confounds this as an outcome measure. The great majority of the information valuable for evaluating DWI treatments is available only from the offender either directly by interview or indirectly through collateral interviews and mechanical measures (e.g., in vehicle monitoring systems). Information on driving practices, accidents, drinking-driving episodes, alcohol consumption, other substance use, and other related measures derived from the offenders must be combined with official information to obtain a convergent view of DWI-related outcomes.

Mandated Assessment and Treatment Is Needed for DWI Offenders

Without mandated assessment, mandated treatment is unlikely to provide the desired results because DWI offenders will seek out programs that may be inappropriate for their constellation of problems. A limited number of assessment domains will be identified as research on DWI treatment-matching matures. Policymakers can utilize these results to produce regulations that require assessment of DWI offenders in the domains that are relevant for treatment matching. The DWI offender would be mandated to complete the most appropriate treatment regimen. This type of system would put an end to treatment shopping and remove the conflict between sanctions and treatment, while giving the highest priority to highway safety and the interests of the general public. However, political realities regarding the time needed to develop new laws and regulations and the need for more guidance from the research literature dictate that it will take some time (in years) before mandated assessment and treatment can be put into place.

Conclusion

This review found reason for optimism for the role of treatment in reducing alcohol-related accidents among DWI offenders. The main reason for this is the potential impact of treatment matching for DWI offenders. Matching efforts specific to the DWI population are justified by:

1. The need to improve DWI intervention outcomes, including accident reduction;
2. The potential shown by alcoholism treatment matching;
3. The recognition of DWI heterogeneity and subgroups;
4. Differential outcomes for DWI offenders using different treatments based on offender severity groups; and
5. The recognition that DWI offenders overlap with the alcoholic population but may require some interventions that alcoholics may not (e.g., driving skills).

Recent findings provide support for the concept that:

1. Treatment can reduce accident-related mortality among DWI offenders;
2. Treatment can potentially impact alcohol-related accident fatalities at a level comparable to other antidrinking-driving approaches; and
3. Treatment can significantly reduce accident-related mortality among DWI offenders.

In addition, the mortality reduction associated with DWI treatment also suggests that treatment benefits outweigh treatment costs. Further, initial reports regarding efforts to reform health care in the United States indicate that substance abuse treatments will be included.[106] This development could further decrease the cost of treatment and enhance the probability of mandated treatment for DWI offenders.

Optimism must be tempered by the fact that even if successful, treatment will be only a part of the answer to alcohol-related accidents and fatalities. In addition, the knowledge base will require years of well-designed research to reach a level where treatment-matching recommendations for DWI offenders can be implemented on a large scale. Nonetheless, this review clearly shows a role for DWI treatment in reducing alcohol-related accidents as part of a comprehensive approach to minimizing drinking and driving and associated problems. The potential contribution of treatment strongly justifies further efforts in this area.

Acknowledgments

This chapter was supported by grants R29AA08920 and K02AA00154 from the National Institute on Alcohol Abuse and Alcoholism. I am also grateful for comments provided by Thomas Nochajski and secretarial assistance provided by Kathy Callanan.

References

[1]P. L. Zador (1991) Alcohol-related relative risk of fatal driver injuries in relation to driver age and sex. *J. Stud. Alcohol* **52,** 302–310.

[2]M. W. Perrine, R. C. Peck, and J. C. Fell (1989) Epidemiologic perspectives on drunken driving, in *Surgeon General's Workshop on Drunk Driving.* US Department of Health and Human Services, Rockville, MD, pp. 36–76.

[3]US Department of Transportation (1984) *Alcohol and Highway Safety 1984: A Review of the State of the Knowledge.* National Highway Traffic Safety Administration, Washington, DC.

[4]US Department of Transportation (1989) *Alcohol and Highway Safety 1984: A Review of the State of the Knowledge.* National Highway Traffic Safety Administration, Washington, DC.

[5]*General Estimates System* (1989) National Highway Traffic Safety Administration, Washington, DC.

[6]J. C. Fell (1990) Drinking and driving in America: disturbing factors—encouraging reductions. *Alcohol Health Res. World* **14(1),** 18–25.

[7]L. Summers and D. Harris (1978) *The General Deterrence of Driving While Intoxicated. Vol 1: System Analysis and Computer-Based Simulation.* Technical Report DOT HS 803 582, National Highway Traffic Safety Administration, Washington, DC.

[8]H. M. Simpson (1985) Human-related risk factors in traffic crashes: research needs and opportunities. *J. Stud. Alcohol* **10,** 32–39.

[9]J. A. Waller (1989) Injury and disability prevention and alcohol-related crashes, in *Surgeon General's Workshop on Drunk Driving.* US Department of Health and Human Services, Rockville, MD, pp. 180–191.

[10]H. L. Ross (1992) *Confronting Drunk Driving: Social Policies for Saving Lives.* Yale University Press, New Haven, CT.

[11]*Surgeon General's Workshop on Drunk Driving* (1989) US Department of Health and Human Services, Rockville, MD.

[12]T. J. Flanagan and K. Maguire (1992) *Sourcebook of Criminal Justice Statistics 1991.* US Department of Justice, Bureau of Justice Statistics, Washington, DC.

[13]E. Vingilis (1983) Drinking drivers and alcoholics: are they from the same population? in *Research Advances in Alcohol and Drug Problems.* R. G. Smart, F. B. Glaser, Y. Israel, H. Kalant, R. E. Popham, and W. Schmidt, eds. Plenum, New York, pp. 299–342.

[14]B. A. Miller and M. Windle (1990) Alcoholism, problem drinking and driving while impaired, in *Drinking and Driving: Advances in Research and Prevention.* R. J. Wilson and R. E. Mann, eds. Guilford, New York, pp. 68–95.

[15]American Psychiatric Association (1987) *Diagnostic and Statistical Manual of Mental Disorders* (3rd ed., rev.). Author, Washington, DC.

[16]W. F. Wieczorek, B. A. Miller, and T. H. Nochajski (1989) *DSM–III and DSM–III–R Alcohol Diagnoses for Problem Drinker Drivers.* Presented at American Psychological Association Convention in New Orleans.

[17]J. E. Helzer and L. N. Robins (1988) The Diagnostic Interview Schedule: its development, evolution, and use. *Soc. Psychiatry Psychiat. Epidemiol.* **23,** 6–16.

[18]W. F. Wieczorek, B. A. Miller, and T. H. Nochajski (1990) Alcohol diagnoses among DWI offenders. *Problem-Drinker Driver Project Research Note, 90-6.*

[19]K. Stewart and V. S. Ellingstad (1989) Rehabilitation countermeasures for drinking drivers, in *Surgeon General's Workshop on Drunk Driving*. US Department of Health and Human Services, Rockville, MD, pp. 234–246.

[20]J. C. Fell (1993) Repeat DWI offenders: their involvement in fatal crashes, in *Alcohol, Drugs and Traffic Safety—92*. H.-D. Utzelmann, G. Berghaus, and G. Kroj, eds. Verlag TUV Rheinland GmbH, Cologne, Germany, pp. 1044–1049.

[21]J. P. M. Bailey (1993) Criminal traffic histories, blood alcohol and accident characteristics of drivers in fatal road accidents in New Zealand, in *Alcohol, Drugs and Traffic Safety—92*. H.-D. Utzelmann, G. Berghaus, and G. Kroj, eds. Verlag TUV Rheinland GmbH, Cologne, Germany, pp. 838–853.

[22]D. S. Reed (1981) Reducing the costs of drinking and driving, in *Alcohol and Public Policy: Beyond the Shadow of Prohibition*. M. H. Moore and D. R. Gerstein, eds. National Academy Press, Washington, DC, pp. 337–387.

[23]A. K. Lund and A. C. Wolf (1991) Changes in the incidence of alcohol-impaired driving in the US, 1973–1986. *J. Stud. Alcohol* **52(4)**, 293–301.

[24]J. L. Nichols (1990) Treatment versus deterrence. *Alcohol Health Res. World* **14(1)**, 44–51.

[25]A. Foon (1988) The effectiveness of drinking-driving treatment programs: a critical review. *Int. J. Addict.* **23**, 151–174.

[26]R. E. Mann, E. R. Vingilis, and K. Stewart (1988) Programs to change individual behavior: education and rehabilitation in the prevention of drinking and driving, in *Social Control of the Drinking Driver*. M. D. Laurence, J. R. Snortum, and F. E. Zimring, eds. The University of Chicago Press, Chicago, pp. 248–269.

[27]E. I. Stewart and J. L. Malfetti (1971) *Rehabilitation of the Drunken Driver: A Corrective Course in Phoenix, Arizona, for Persons Convicted of Driving Under the Influence of Alcohol*. Teachers College Press, New York.

[28]H. A. Siegal (1985) *Impact of a Driver Intervention Program on DWI Recidivism and Problem Drinking*. Department of Transportation, Washington, DC.

[29]R. B. Voas and A. S. Tippets (1990) Evaluation of treatment and monitoring programs for drunken drivers. *J. Traffic Med.* **18**, 15–26.

[30]R. Washousky (1986) An alcoholic outpatient treatment program for alcoholics convicted of DWI, in *Stop DWI*. D. Foley ed. Heath, Lexington, MA, pp. 77–83.

[31]W. F. Wieczorek (1993) Treatment histories of severe DWI offenders, in *Alcohol, Drugs and Traffic Safety—92*. H.-D. Utzelmann, G. Berghaus, and G. Kroj, eds. Verlag TUV Rheinland GmbH, Cologne, Germany, pp. 305–310.

[32]J. L. Fitzgerald (1992) Problems in the evaluation of treatment programs for drunk drivers: goals and outcomes. *J. Drug Iss.* **22(1)**, 155–167.

[33]R. E. Mann, G. Leigh, E. R. Vingilis, and K. De Genova (1983) A critical review on the effectiveness of drinking-driving rehabilitation programs. *Accident Anal. Prev.* **15(6)**, 441–461.

[34]R. B. Voas (1981) Results and implications of the ASAPS, in *Alcohol, Drugs, and Traffic Safety, Vol. 3*. L. Goldberg ed. Almqvist & Wiksell International, Stockholm, pp. 1129–1144.

[35]J. L. Nichols, E. B. Weinstein, V. S. Ellingstad, and R. E. Reis (1981) The effectiveness of education and treatment programs for drinking drivers: a decade of evaluation, in *Alcohol, Drugs, and Traffic Safety, Vol. 3*. L. Goldberg ed. Almqvist & Wiksell International, Stockholm, Sweden, pp. 1298–1328.

[36]V. S. Ellingstad and D L. Struckman-Johnson (1978) *Short Term Rehabilitation (STR) Study: 12 Month Analysis.* National Highway Traffic Safety Administration, Washington, DC.

[37]V. S. Ellingstad and D. L. Struckman-Johnson (1978) *Short Term Rehabilitation (STR) Study: 18 Month Analysis.* National Highway Traffic Safety Administration, Washington, DC.

[38]R. A. Brown (1980) Conventional education and controlled drinking education courses with convicted drunken drivers. *Behav. Ther.* **11**, 632–642.

[39]R. A. Brown (1980) Knowledge about responsible drinking in drinking drivers and social drinkers. *Int. J. Addict.* **15(8)**, 1213–1218.

[40]J. L. Nichols (1979) The effectiveness of ASAP education and rehabilitation programs, in *Proceedings: Seventh International Conference on Alcohol, Drugs and Traffic Safety, 1977.* I. R. Johnson, ed. Australian Government Publishing Service, Canberra, Australia, pp. 622–629.

[41]E. Vingilis, E. Adlaf, and L. Chung (1981) The Oshawa impaired drivers programme: an evaluation of a rehabilitation programme. *Can. J. Criminol.* **23(1)**, 93–102.

[42]W. F. Blount, R. E. Reis, Jr., and J. E. Chappell (1983) The effects of drinking driver rehabilitation efforts on rearrests when drinker type is controlled, in *DWI Reeducation and Rehabilitation Programs.* AAA Foundation for Traffic Safety, Falls Church, VA, pp. 22–37.

[43]D. W. Essex and W. B. Weinerth (1982) *Effects of Treatment on the DUI Offender in Ventura County.* Alcohol Services Program, Health Care Agency, Ventura, CA.

[44]R. Holden (1983) Rehabilitative sanctions for drunk driving: an experimental evaluation. *J. Res. Crime Delinq.* **20**, 55–72.

[45]J. Landrum, S. Miles, R. Neff, T. Pritchard, J. Roebuck, E. Wells-Parker, and G. Windham (1982) *Mississippi DUI Probation Follow-Up Project.* National Highway Traffic Safety Administration, Washington, DC.

[46]E. Wells-Parker, B. J. Anderson, J. W. Landrum, and R. W. Snow (1988) Long-term effectiveness of probation, short-term intervention and LAI administration for reducing DUI recidivism. *Br. J. Addict.* **83**, 415–421.

[47]R. E. Reis, Jr. (1980) *First Interim Analysis of First Offender Treatment Effectiveness.* National Highway Traffic Safety Administration, Washington, DC.

[48]R. E. Reis, Jr. (1983) The traffic safety impact of DWI education and counseling programs, in *DWI Reeducation and Rehabilitation Programs.* AAA Foundation for Traffic Safety, Falls Church, VA, pp. 38–61.

[49]F. L. McGuire (1982) Treatment of the drinking driver. *Health Psychol.* **1**, 137–152.

[50]J. L. Nichols, V. S. Ellingstad, and D. L. Struckman-Johnson (1979) An experimental evaluation of the effectiveness of short-term education and rehabilitation programs for convicted drinking drivers, in *Currents in Alcoholism: Treatment and Rehabilitation and Epidemiology.* M. Galanter ed. Grune & Stratton, New York, pp. 157–177.

[51]H. A. Siegal and P. A. Cole (1993) Enhancing criminal justice based treatment through the application of the intervention approach. *J. Drug Issues* **23(2)**, 131–142.

[52]D. M. Donovan, P. M. Salzberg, E. F. Chaney, H. R. Queisser, and G. A. Marlatt (1989) Prevention skills for alcohol-involved drivers. *Alcohol, Drugs, Driving* **6(3–4)**, 169–188.

[53]T. H. Nochajski, B. A. Miller, W. F. Wieczorek, and R. Whitney (1993) The effects of a drinker-driver treatment program: does criminal history make a difference? *Crim. Just. Behav.* **20(2)**, 174–189.

[54]R. E. Mann, L. Anglin, K. Wilkins, E. R. Vingilis, S. MacDonald, and W. J. Sheu (1994) Rehabilitation for convicted drinking drivers (second offense): effects on mortality. *J. Stud. Alcohol* **55(3)**, 372–374.

[55]D. Donovan (1989) Driving while intoxicated: different roads to and from the problem. *Crim. Just. Behav.* **16,** 270–298.

[56]R. E. Mann (1992) Effectiveness of DUI treatment and the importance of screening and matching clients to appropriate treatment, in *Drinking and Driving Prevention Symposium.* Automobile Club of Southern California, Ontario, CA, pp. 129–145.

[57]E. Wells-Parker, J. W. Landrum, and J. S. Topping (1990) Matching the DWI offender to an effective intervention strategy: an emerging research agenda, in *Drinking and Driving: Advances in Research and Prevention.* R. J. Wilson and R. E. Mann, eds. Guilford, New York, pp. 267–289.

[58]W. F. Wieczorek and B. A. Miller (1992) Preliminary typology designed for treatment matching of DWI offenders. *J. Consult. Clin. Psychol.* **60(5),** 757–765.

[59]D. M. Donovan and D. Rosengren (1992) Effectiveness of alcohol treatment and treatment matching: how DUI treatment may be improved by insights from the alcoholism treatment field, in *Drinking and Driving Prevention Symposium.* Automobile Club of Southern California, Ontario, CA, pp. 129–145.

[60]K. M. Bowman and E. M. Jellinek (1941) Alcohol addiction and its treatment. *Q. J. Stud. Alcohol* **2,** 98–176.

[61]H. M. Annis (1987) *Effective Treatment for Drug and Alcohol Problems: What Do We Know?* Presented at the annual meeting of the Institute of Medicine, National Academy of Sciences, Washington, DC.

[62]J. W. Finney and R. H. Moos (1986) Matching patients with treatments: conceptual and methodological issues. *J. Stud. Alcohol* **47(2),** 122–134.

[63]W. R. Miller (1989) Matching individuals with interventions, in *Handbook of Alcoholism Treatment Approaches,* R. K. Hester and W. R. Miller eds. Pergamon, New York, pp. 261–271.

[64]Committee to Identify Research Opportunities in the Prevention and Treatment of Alcohol-Related Problems (1992) Prevention and treatment of alcohol-related problems: research opportunities. *J. Stud. Alcohol* **53(1),** 5–16.

[65]W. R. Miller and R. K. Hester (1986) Matching problem drinkers with optimal treatments, in *Treating Addictive Behaviors: Processes of Change.* W. R. Miller and N. Heather, eds. Plenum, New York, pp. 175–203.

[66]J. Orford, E. Oppenheimer, and G. Edwards (1976) Abstinence or control: the outcome for excessive drinkers two years after consultation. *Behav. Res. Ther.* **14,** 409–418.

[67]M. D. Litt, F. Del Boca, N. L. Cooney, R. M. Kadden, and T. Babor (1989) Matching alcoholics to aftercare treatment by empirical clustering: predicting relapse. *Alcohol Clin. Exp.* **13(2),** 350.

[68]B. J. Rounsaville, Z. S. Dolinsky, T. F. Babor, and R. E. Meyer (1987) Psychopathology as a predictor of treatment outcome in alcoholics. *Arch. Gen. Psychiatry* **44,** 505–513.

[69]A. T. McLellan, L. Luborsky, G. E. Woody, and C. P. O'Brien (1980). An improved diagnostic evaluation instrument for substance abuse patients: the Addiction Severity Index. *J. Nervous Mental Dis.* **168,** 26–33.

[70]A. T. McLellan, G. E. Woody, L. Luborsky, C. P. O'Brien, and K. A. Druley (1983) Increased effectiveness of substance abuse treatment. *J. Nervous Mental Dis.* **171(10),** 597–605.

[71]R. M. Kadden, N. L. Cooney, H. Getter, and M. D. Litt (1989) Matching alcoholics to coping skills or interactional therapies: posttreatment results. *J. Consult. Clin. Psychol.* **57(6),** 698–704.

[72]J. F. C. McLachlan (1972) Benefit from group therapy as a function of patient–therapist match on conceptual level. *Psychotherapy* **9,** 317–323.

[73]J. F. C. McLachlan (1974) Therapy strategies, personality orientation and recovery from alcoholism. *Can. Psychiat. Assoc. J.* **19,** 25–30.

[74]H. M. Annis and D. Chan (1983) The differential treatment model: empirical evidence from a personality typology of adult offenders. *Crim. Just. Behav.* **10(2),** 159–173.

[75]D. J. Armor, J. M. Polich, and H. B. Stambul (1978) *Alcoholism and Treatment.* Wiley, New York.

[76]N. H. Azrin, R. W. Sisson, R. Meyers, and M. Godley (1982) Alcoholism treatment by disulfiram and community reinforcement therapy. *Behav. Ther. Exp. Psychiatry* **13,** 105–112.

[77]T. F. Babor, Z. S. Dolinsky, R. E. Meyer, M. Hesselbrock, M. Hofmann, and H. Tennen (1992) Types of alcoholics: concurrent and predictive validity of some common classification schemes. *Br. J. Addict.* **87,** 1415–1431.

[78]T. F. Babor, M. Hofmann, F K. DelBoca, V. Hesselbrock, R. E. Meyer, Z. S. Dolinsky, and B. Rounsaville (1992) Types of alcoholics, I. Evidence for an empirically derived typology based on indicators of vulnerability and severity. *Arch. Gen. Psychiatry* **49,** 599–608.

[79]M. D. Litt, T. F. Babor, F. K. DelBoca, R. M. Kadden, and N. L. Cooney (1992) Applications of an empirically derived typology to treatment matching. *Arch. Gen. Psychiatry* **49,** 609–614.

[80]H. Moskowitz, J. Walker, and C. Gomberg (1979) Characteristics of DWIs, alcoholics and controls, in *Proceedings of the 1979 NCA Alcohol and Traffic Safety Session.* National Highway Traffic Safety Administration, Washington, DC, pp. 9–79.

[81]M. W. Perrine (1975) Alcohol, drugs, and driving: relative priorities for basic and applied research, in *Alcohol, Drugs and Traffic Safety.* S. Israelstam and S. Lambert, eds. Addiction Research Foundation, Toronto, pp. 107–128.

[82]E. A. Pristach, T. H. Nochajski, W. F. Wieczorek, B. A. Miller, and B. Greene (1991) Psychiatric symptoms and DWI offenders. *Alcohol & Alcoholism* **1,** 493–496.

[83]D. L. McMillen, M. G. Pang, E. Wells-Parker, and B. J. Anderson (1992) Alcohol, personality traits, and high risk driving: a comparison of young, drinking driver groups. *Addict. Behav.* **17,** 525–532.

[84]D. Donovan (1980) *Drinking Behavior, Personality Factors and High-Risk Driving.* Unpublished doctoral dissertation, University of Washington, Seattle.

[85]M. Argeriou, D. McCarty, and E. Blacker (1985) Criminality among individuals arraigned for drinking and driving in Massachusetts. *J. Stud. Alcohol* **46(6),** 525–530.

[86]G. W. Lucker, D. J. Kruzich, and M. T. Holt (1991) The prevalence of antisocial behavior among U.S. Army DWI offenders. *J. Stud. Alcohol* **52(4)**, 318–320.

[87]S. MacDonald (1989) A comparison of the psychosocial characteristics of alcoholics responsible for impaired and nonimpaired collisions. *Accid. Anal. Prev.* **21(5)**, 493–508.

[88]S. MacDonald and L. L. Pederson (1988) Occurrence and patterns of driving behaviour for alcoholics in treatment. *Drug Alcohol Depend.* **22**, 15–25.

[89]D. M. Donovan, H. R. Queisser, P. M. Salzberg, and R. L. Umlauf (1985) Intoxicated and bad drivers: subgroups within the same population of high-risk men drivers. *J. Stud. Alcohol* **46(5)**, 375–382.

[90]D. M. Donovan, R. L. Umlauf, and P. M. Salzberg (1990) Bad drivers: identification of a target group for alcohol-related prevention and early intervention. *J. Stud. Alcohol* **51(2)**, 136–141.

[91]G. W. Arstein-Kerslake and R. C. Peck (1985) *A Typological Analysis of California DUI Offenders and DUI Recidivism Correlates.* NTIS No. DOT-HS-806-994, National Highway Traffic Safety Administration, Department of Transportation, Washington, DC.

[92]D. M. Donovan and G. A. Marlatt (1982) Personality subtypes among driving-while-intoxicated offenders: relationship to drinking behavior and driving risk. *J. Consult. Clin. Psychol.* **50(2)**, 242–249.

[93]R. L. Snowden, L. S. Nelson, and D. Campbell (1986) An empirical typology of problem drinkers from the Michigan Alcoholism Screening Test. *Addict. Behav.* **11**, 37–48.

[94]R. A. Steer, E. W. Fine, and P. E. Scholes (1979) Classification of men arrested for driving while intoxicated and treatment implications: a cluster-analytic study. *J. Stud. Alcohol* **40**, 222–229.

[95]E. Wells-Parker, P. J. Cosby, and J. W. Landrum (1986) A typology for drinking driving offenders: methods for classification and policy implications. *Accident Anal. Prev.* **18**, 443–453.

[96]R. J. Wilson (1991) Subtypes of DWIs and high risk drivers: implications for differential intervention. *Alcohol, Drugs, Driving* **7(1)**, 1–12.

[97]D. M. Donovan, D. R. Kivlahan, and R. D. Walker (1986) Alcoholic subtypes based on multiple assessment domains validation against treatment outcome, in *Recent Developments in Alcoholism, Vol. 4.* M. Galanter ed. Plenum, New York, pp. 207–222.

[98]E. Wells-Parker, B. Anderson, and M. Pang (1993) An examination of cluster-based classification schemes for DUI offenders. *J. Stud. Alcohol* **54**, 209–218.

[99]R. K. Blashfield (1984) *The Classification of Psychopathology. Neo-Kraepelinian and Quantitative Approaches.* Plenum, New York.

[100]G. W. Milligan and M. C. Cooper (1987) Methodology review: clustering methods. *Appl. Psychol. Meas.* **11(4)**, 329–354.

[101]D. M. Donovan, G. A. Marlatt, and P. M. Salzberg (1983) Drinking behavior, personality factors and high-risk driving. *J. Stud. Alcohol* **44(3)**, 395–428.

[102]D. D. Sadler and M. L. W. Perrine (1984) *The Long Term Traffic Safety Impact of a Pilot Alcohol Abuse Treatment as an Alternative to License Suspension.* California Department of Motor Vehicles, Sacramento, CA.

[103]R. C. Peck, D. D. Sadler, and M. W. Perrine (1985) The comparative effectiveness of alcohol rehabilitation and licensing control actions for drunk driving offenders: a review of the literature. *Alcohol, Drugs, Driving* **1(4),** 15–39.

[104]R. E. Mann and E. R. Vingilis (1989) Assessment issues in problem drinking and rehabilitation outcome, in *Alcohol, Drugs and Traffic Safety.* Proceedings of the 11th International Conference on Alcohol, Drugs and Traffic Safety, National Safety Council, Chicago, pp. 184–188.

[105]D. M. Donovan (1989) Subtypes among risk and drunk drivers: implications for assessment, and rehabilitation, in *Alcohol, Drugs and Traffic Safety.* Proceedings of the 11th International Conference on Alcohol, Drugs and Traffic Safety, National Safety Council, Chicago, pp. 184–188.

[106]A reader's guide to health reform (September 20, 1993) *Newsweek,* pp. 34,35.

Review of the Effects
of the Alcohol Warning Label

David P. MacKinnon

Introduction

Warning labels on alcohol containers were proposed as early as 1945.[1] In 1988, legislation was passed requiring the following warning label on alcoholic beverage containers beginning on November 18, 1989.[2]

> GOVERNMENT WARNING: (1) According to the Surgeon General, women should not drink alcoholic beverages during pregnancy because of the risk of birth defects. (2) Consumption of alcoholic beverages impairs your ability to drive a car or operate machinery, and may cause health problems.

The purpose of this chapter is to review research on the effects of the alcohol warning label and relevant research on alcohol warning posters and proposed warnings on alcohol advertisements. Warning labels are described in the context of other methods to prevent alcohol abuse. The effects of warnings similar to the alcohol warning are described. Models for how the alcohol warning label might work and the goals and major criticisms of warnings are discussed. The main findings of natural and deliberate experiments are summarized and directions for future research are suggested.

Problem

The economic and health costs of alcohol abuse are substantial because of its involvement in a wide range of health and social problems: cancer, cardiovascular disease, homicide, drownings, automobile accidents, and accidents at work.[3] Each year approx 20,000 traffic fatalities and a quarter

From: *Drug and Alcohol Abuse Reviews, Vol. 7: Alcohol, Cocaine, and Accidents*
Ed.: R. R. Watson ©1995 Humana Press Inc., Totowa, NJ

of a million traffic injuries involve alcohol.[4] Approximately 1500 babies are born each year with Fetal Alcohol Syndrome (FAS), which is characterized by severe mental and physical birth defects caused by the pregnant mother's alcohol use.[5]

Warning Labels as an Alcohol Prevention Strategy

Many different types of preventive interventions have been implemented in an attempt to reduce alcohol-related problems. These include limiting access or availability,[6,7] increasing the sales tax,[8,9] raising the drinking age,[10–12] increasing the severity and certainty of punishment,[13–15] and school- and community-based alcohol prevention programs.[16–18] Although there is evidence that each of these efforts has had at least some success (especially taxation and drinking age changes), some effects have been temporary (e.g., drunk driving deterrents) and others have been labor intensive and limited in dissemination (e.g., school and community programs).

Mass media-based intervention could provide an alternative or a complement to prevention programs. However, relatively little is known about the capability of mass media for producing sustained changes in drinking behavior. Results of prior research on advertising effects are controversial and ambiguous, with some studies suggesting an effect, and other studies showing no effect on attitudinal or behavioral change.[19–21] Reviews of research in this area suggest that mass media interventions have the capacity to change drug use by first changing attitudes toward drug use.[22] Mass media may also cultivate certain attitudes and behaviors that take several years to change behavior.[23] Other interventions, such as school and community programs, may increase the impact of mass media interventions by cuing audiences to select and attend to the mass media message.[24]

Alcohol warning labels may represent a low-cost media intervention effective by itself or as a cue to school and other prevention activities. The warning provides information only and does not directly place constraints on behavior. Warning labels have considerable public support and the risks mentioned on the label are viewed as serious public health problems by the majority of citizens.[25] Because the warning is on all alcoholic beverages, alcohol consumers are repeatedly exposed to it. Furthermore, the potential exposure to the warning increases as alcohol use increases, thereby warning the group most likely at risk.

Goals of the Alcohol Warning Label

There are different perspectives on the goals of warning labels. (*See* refs. 26 and 27 for comprehensive discussions of warning labels.) The text of the law states that the purpose of the alcohol warning label is to inform and remind the public about the risks of alcohol use and to reduce uncertainty and misperceptions about alcohol use consequences. As is described later, in the majority of research studies, most persons are aware of the risks on the alcohol warning, except perhaps for the risk of birth defects. Some researchers suggest that the primary purpose of the warning is to increase public perception of the risk of alcohol use,[28] but perceptions of negative consequences are not always substantial predictors of consumption or problems with alcohol.[29]

Changing behavior is not directly mentioned in the text of the law, although changing behavior is often cited as the ultimate criterion of the effectiveness of warnings.[30] Whether warnings change behavior is controversial,[31-33] and the beneficial effects of the alcohol warning label have also been questioned.[34-38] The ultimate criterion for alcohol misuse prevention strategies is a change in the incidence and prevalence of alcohol-related problems. The alcohol warning may act in combination with other alcohol abuse prevention strategies to reduce alcohol-related problems.

From a legal perspective, warnings are viewed as a cost-effective strategy to inform and instruct consumers in the proper use of a product.[27] Manufacturers satisfy their "duty to warn" and they receive some limitation of liability.[39] The general attitude among many legal and other professionals is always to warn because it informs users and protects the manufacturers.[40-44]

Criticisms of the Alcohol Warning Label

The alcohol warning label has been criticized because persons are already aware of the risks of alcohol use and too many warnings may divert attention from critical warnings.[27,45-47] Driver[45] stated that "Warning labels should be reserved for only those products where it can be determined that labels will be an effective means of communication and will not be harmful" (p. 163). A widely used human factors textbook[48] concludes that "From a human factors perspective, excessive warnings are as bad as insufficient warnings. People become accustomed to the warnings and tend to ignore them" (p. 634). Further, Weinstein et al.[46] asserted that "One must warn discriminantly if one expects the [user] to heed the warning" (p. 63). Although there is theoretical support for the notion of overwarning, there does not appear to be substantial empirical research on the effects of overwarning.

Information on the effects of multiple warnings may be drawn from studies of message repetition. Cacioppo and Petty[49,50] studied the effects of message repetition on recall and comprehension of message information. Moderate repetition of a message "is posited to result in a greater realization of the meaning, interconnections, and implications of the messages' arguments. . . ." (p. 4).[50] In the case of warnings, this would suggest that a moderately repeated warning would be beneficial to processing the content of the warnings. During high levels of message-repetition, psychological reactance occurs analogous to the overwarning effect.

A process by which overwarning may occur is suggested by the psychological processes operating when persons are warned of a threat but do not experience any negative consequences.[51] As in Aesop's fable. "The Boy and the Wolf," if threats are made without negative consequences, there is a loss in the credibility of the source of the warning and protective action is less likely to be taken. The effect, called the False Alarm Effect,[52] may also explain the familiarity effect in human factors research[53,54] where persons perceive products as less harmful and are less likely to read a warning as they become more familiar with them. If alcohol users see the warnings repeatedly, yet never experience any negative outcomes with the product, then the warning may lose credibility and protective action may be less likely.

Theory and Models for the Effects of Warning Labels

Several theories provide guidance for how the alcohol warning label may influence behavior. All of these theories predict that behavior change may result from small changes over a long period, and immediate effects on behavior are unlikely.

McGuire's Stages of Communication

McGuire's[55] communication model is the most cited model in alcohol warning research.[56–59] In this model, there are 10 successive steps necessary for effective health risk communication/persuasion. According to the model, a person must:

1. See the label;
2. Attend to the label;
3. React affectively to it;
4. Comprehend the risk information;
5. Agree or yield to the material;
6. Store and retain the content of the warning;
7. Search and retrieve the information when needed;
8. Make a decision based on the warning;
9. Behave on the basis of that decision; and
10. Consolidate the behavior so that the behavior will occur on other occasions.

The effects of warning labels on actual behavior are small because each of the successive steps must be passed for the label to change behavior. The theory indicates that the evaluation of warning labels must include measures of intermediate processes such as source, memory, and various social and personality characteristics. The model suggests a linear Guttman scale through the steps toward changing behavior.

McGuire's model was slightly modified by Lehto and Miller[27] to include eight steps. These authors note that a linear sequence may not be accurate. The possibility that the steps can be skipped or the existence of indirect as well as direct paths among the measures does not appear to have been empirically tested.

The Health Belief Model

The Health Belief Model[60] suggests that the likelihood of preventive health behavior increases as perceived threat increases and as the ratio of perceived benefits to perceived costs associated with taking that action also increases. Perceived threat is comprised of the person's perceived susceptibility to the negative outcome associated with not taking the preventive action, and the perceived severity or seriousness of that outcome. The theory suggests that information available at the time the person will be making the health-related decision greatly increases the likelihood that the preventive action will be taken. This information, called cues to action in the model, increases the amount of threat the person feels regarding the potential negative outcome. In a review of the health belief model, Janz and Becker[60] concluded, "Unfortunately, few Health Belief Model studies have attempted to assess the contribution of 'cues' to predicting health actions" (p. 3).

The alcohol warning label may serve as a cue to avoid alcohol.[57,61] The warning label may cue the risks of alcohol use by making them more accessible in memory, especially when alcohol is consumed. Recent theory about the effects of alcohol-related beliefs on alcohol use suggest that these risks affect behavior only if they "come to mind" in drinking situations.[62–65] In the expectancy-accessibility model of alcohol,[29] for example, beliefs about risks affect behavior only if they are accessed during drinking decisions.

Advertising Theory Model

Leckenby and Plummer[66] proposed a model for testing advertisements based on cognitive and affective learning. In this model, warning labels can have a variety of effects other than the cognitive change that is the focus of the other two models. There are six different levels of advertising stimulus measurement in the model:

1. Preconscious response;
2. Concurrent affective response;
3. Immediate cognitive response;
4. Retained cognitive response;
5. Immediate behavioral response; and
6. Delayed behavioral response.

This model suggests that affective or emotional reactions to the warning may also lead to behavior change or persuasion. As an example, cognitive processing of the label may suggest other meanings of the warning label, e.g., the government deems that labels are necessary, which may induce a norm more negative toward alcohol misuse.

Effects of Tobacco Warnings

The impact of cigaret and smokeless tobacco warning labels provide information to anticipate or understand the effects of alcohol warning labels. All are addictive substances recognized as risk factors for premature death. Because cigaret labels were introduced 1 yr after the Surgeon General's report[67] and improved in 1970 during the antismoking advertising campaign, the effects of the legislation on consumption and problems were not distinguishable from the effects of other antismoking activity.[68,69] Laboratory research on the cigaret warning suggests that it is believable,[70] changing the warning can affect memory[71] and advertisements with warnings are less attractive and less persuasive.[72] In laboratory studies, a relatively small percentage of persons view the warning in billboard or magazine advertisements.[73,74] Smokeless tobacco warnings are also believable,[75] but may not be noticeable,[76] although users do appear to have more accurate memory for the label than nonusers.[77] A consistent conclusion from the tobacco warnings research was that it was a missed opportunity to learn about the effects of warning labels.

Unlike cigaret warning labels, alcohol labels appeared after major alcohol prevention activity began in the late 1970s.[78] Strategies to reduce alcohol consumption are not increasing rapidly,[79,80] although the social norm may be becoming less tolerant of alcohol misuse. Alcohol labeling effects may also differ from the effects of cigaret labels because problems owing to alcohol use are more immediate (e.g., impaired driving vs lung cancer) and the warning label is on the alcohol container (when drinking out of the can or bottle) not the packaging, as for cigarets.

Studies Included in the Review

The National Institute on Alcoholism and Alcohol Abuse funded several projects[81] to study the effects of the alcohol warning label and several other researchers have conducted unfunded or partially funded research on the warning label. In a review of the effects of the alcohol warning label, Hilton[57] concluded that awareness of the label has increased, but there is little or no evidence for an effect on perceptions of risk or behaviors targeted by the warning. I have tried to supplement Hilton's review by describing both deliberate studies and natural experiments used to examine the effects of the alcohol warning label, alcohol warning posters, and proposed warnings on alcohol advertisements. Many studies have also been published or accepted for publication since Hilton's review.

Deliberate studies are designed to examine some aspect of the warning using either randomization or observational methods. None of the deliberate studies include measures both before and after the label was introduced. Natural experiments are studies of the effects of the warning label and warning poster where implementation of the intervention (the warning label or poster) was not under investigator control but both prelabel and postlabel measures were available. There have been natural experiments on the effects of the warning label and warning poster, but not warnings or advertisements, as the proposal requiring warnings on advertisements has not become law.

I attempted to obtain all alcohol warning studies by contacting authors by mail or phone and through literature searches. Research on the effect of the alcohol warning through 1992 were available, so the review reflects 3-yr effects of the label. Only published and in press articles or university technical reports are included. The articles fall in a relatively wide range of journals reflecting authors from a variety of disciplines, including public policy and marketing, human factors, law, public health, and psychology.

Deliberate Studies

Deliberate studies of alcohol warnings are summarized in Table 1. The majority of the studies have been conducted in laboratory settings using college students as subjects. The studies are organized by the topic studied.

Noticeability of the Container Label

Laughery and colleagues[82] conducted three experiments on the noticeability of the alcohol warning label. Subjects were recruited by telephone and were sampled to reflect the adult population based on ethnic group, gender, and age. (Age was not used to sample subjects in Experiment 3.) Noticeability was measured as the speed to notice that there was a warning on a container. Each subject responded to all containers, of which some had labels. The overall conclusion from these experiments was that warnings on the containers were not particularly noticeable, primarily because the warnings do not stand out from their background. In Experiment 1, label clutter, vertical placement, and placement other than the front of the container made the warning less noticeable. In Experiments 2 and 3, pictorials, icons, and color improved the noticeability of the warning, whereas borders did not have much effect. Pictorials appeared to produce

Table 1
Deliberate Studies of Alcohol Warnings

Studies	Sample	Method	Measures
Andrews et al. (1991, 1993)[86-88]	College students (N = 273)	Questionnaire	Believability
Barlow and Wogalter (1993)[90]	College students (N = 105, 120)	Presentation of warning in a magazine advertisement and in commercials during a basketball game	Recall and recognition
Godfrey et al. (1992)[83]	Adults (N = 60)	Presentation of warnings in different location	Time to locate the warning
Kalsher et al. (1993)	College fraternity members (N = 134, 84)	Exposure to alcohol facts poster	Knowledge
Laughery et al. (1993)[82]	Adults (N = 75, 72, 24)	Presentation of warning in different locations on the bottle	Time to locate the warning
MacKinnon et al. (1992)[85]	College students (N = 288)	Presentation of the label and memory tests	Memory measures
MacKinnon et al. (1993)[77]	College students (N = 288, 243)	Questionnaire	Memory, drug use
MacKinnon et al. (1993)[91]	College students (N = 111, 75)	Choice-based scenario	Choice
MacKinnon et al. (1994)[92]	College and high school students (N = 292, 813, 145)	Choice-based scenario	Avoidance of labels
Malouff et al. (1993)[84]	Bar patrons and college students (N = 44, 50, 44, 75)	Cued to warning or not	Conspicuousness ratings, recall, alcohol use
Smith (1990)[89]	College students (N = 445)	Manipulated severity of the warning and mode of presentation	Recall and beliefs
Snyder and Blood (1992)[28]	College students (N = 159)	Advertisements with and without warnings	Perception of risks and benefits

the most substantial effects. There was evidence that combining features may increase the noticeability but in a complex way; e.g., the addition of an icon produced a significant improvement in performance but only when colored black, not red.

Two other studies replicated the positive effect of horizontal rather than vertical labels. Using a similar experimental procedure to the afore-mentioned studies Godfrey et al.[83] also found that horizontal warnings and warnings on the front of the containers were more quickly identified. Less clutter and the "Government Warning" phrase also reduced response times. The horizontal warning was rated more conspicuous than the vertical warning and the container with a horizontal label led to more accurate memory than a vertical label in another study.[84]

Effects of Processing
on Memory for the Container Label

MacKinnon et al.[85] hypothesized that the warning label may be pro-cessed in three ways:

1. Persons may read the label;
2. Persons may read the label and describe its contents to others; and
3. Persons may see the label but not cognitively process the label.

Processing effects were operationalized as three orienting tasks to the label (read, paraphrase, and count), which were compared to a control condition (no experimental exposure to the warning label). Four tests (free recall, recognition, word-stem completion, and controlled association) were compared. In one additional condition, subjects were cued to the warning label without prior experimental exposure. The free recall test was the most sensitive measure to different levels of processing. Average memory scores for the paraphrase and read conditions were higher than the count and control conditions. Average memory performance in the cued condition was superior to the control condition, suggesting that subjects remem-ber the content of the warning from exposure to the label outside the experiment.

Effects of Cuing the Container Label

Malouff et al.[84] conducted an experimental study of prompting atten-tion to the warning label in a Florida bar. Seventy-five bar patrons were randomly assigned to either a control or experimental group. Subjects in the experimental group were approached by an experimenter who asked, "Did you notice whether there was a warning on the can (bottle) you just had?" and if the warning was noticed they were asked, "How much of the warning can you remember?" After both cued and control patrons left the bar, their written bill was obtained and the number of drinks counted. Patrons who were prompted drank significantly fewer drinks (3.56 vs 4.30). Among the treatment group subjects, greater recall for the warning label was asso-ciated with less alcohol use ($r = -.39$).

Alcohol Use and Memory for the Container Label

Measures of substance use and recognition memory for warning labels were collected from college students.[77] It was hypothesized that if health warnings were noticed and remembered, then users, because they were often exposed to the warning labels, would have more accurate memory for the risks written on the containers of these products than nonusers. A statistically significant correlation was obtained between use and recognition memory for cigarets, smokeless tobacco, and alcohol use. As alcohol use increased, recognition memory increased, suggesting that alcohol users do process the content of the label to an extent that it improves memory. The results were replicated in a sample of high school students.[58]

Attitudes Toward and Believability of Advertisement Warnings

Andrews et al.[86] studied believability and attitudes about the five warnings proposed for alcohol advertisements, several of which appear on the alcohol warning label. The warning of the risk of birth defects was the most believable warning. The risk of impaired driving was more believable than the other warnings—risk of hypertension, liver disease, and cancer; addictive; and dangerous if used in combination with other drugs. Attitudes toward the birth defects warning were more favorable than the other warnings, which were all equally favorable. Alcohol users were less likely to believe the risks.[87]

In another article based on the same data, Andrews et al.[88] conducted a mediation analysis of measures that were part of the experimental manipulation. Subjects listed the thoughts that came to mind after reading each warning label. A measure of net support (support for the label minus arguments against the label) mediated the relationship between attitude toward drinking and attitude toward each warning label.

Experimental Studies of Advertisement Warnings

Smith[89] reviewed the effects of warnings in advertisements and then examined advertisements that varied on the severity of the warning, type of presentation (video or radio), and relevance of the product. After a median split on alcohol consumption, undergraduate college students were randomized into one of six conditions defined by presentation (video, audio, or audio-video), severity (high or low), or one of two control groups (no warning or different advertisement). The dependent variables were aided and unaided recall, and product safety beliefs based on Likert-scale type items.

A majority of subjects recalled the advertisement without aid. Of the subjects exposed to a warning message, 36.2% recalled a warning disclosure of some type and 21% accurately recalled the warning message without aid. Audio presentation led to the greatest overall recall and video presentation led to the poorest recall. Subjects who saw a more severe warning had more accurate recall. There were no significant differences among the conditions on product safety beliefs.

Barlow and Wogalter[90] examined the effects of magazine and television advertisements. More conspicuous warnings on the print adds led to better memory and knowledge in Experiment 1. Both voice and on-screen warnings led to the greatest memory, and students in the print only condition performed as well as subjects in both modality conditions. The authors concluded that simultaneous audio and video presentation is the best method to present warnings in television commercials. The warnings in these experiments were not identical to the proposed media or alcohol warning label.

Snyder and Blood[28] concluded that warnings on alcohol advertisements may be counterproductive for some subjects. Undergraduates were randomly assigned to one of four conditions. Subjects older than 22 yr were eliminated from the study. The experiment was conducted in April 1990 and October 1990 after the warning label had been required to appear on alcoholic beverages. Subjects were shown slides of six different alcohol products. The slides were viewed with and without a warning in four conditions:

1. A slide of a bottle of alcohol;
2. The Surgeon General's warning at the bottom;
3. A bottle in a magazine advertisement without a warning; and
4. A bottle in a magazine advertisement with a warning at the bottom.

The dependent variables were scales of alcohol product benefits, alcohol product risks, risks suggested by the warnings in the experiment, and social risks. Alcohol use and gender were confounded, such that there were only four male nondrinkers who were not included in the analysis.

The advertisement and warning had no effect on the social alcohol risk or the personal alcohol risk measures. Viewing the advertisements led to higher benefit ratings and lower risk ratings, especially among nondrinkers (all females). Warnings had no effect on product risk perception, and the nondrinkers (all females) had lower benefit estimates when exposed to the warnings. In contrast, drinkers had greater benefit estimates when the warning was present. Male drinkers who viewed the advertisements with warnings had greater drinking intentions compared to female drinkers and female nondrinkers.

Avoidance Responses to Alternative Warnings

MacKinnon and colleagues[91,92] used a choice-based method to compare alternative warning labels, including the existing alcohol warning label, warnings proposed for advertisements, and earlier proposed warnings. The purpose of this research was to explore the extent to which certain labels elicit an avoidance response. In two studies using a questionnaire format, a "poison," "toxic," or "causes cancer" label on a beer can was shown to have substantial effects on self-reported choice behavior. In contrast, the alcohol warning label now mandated to appear on alcohol containers did not have nearly as powerful an effect. In three other studies among college and high school students, it was found that specific risks were more important than the overall label length, qualifier words such as "may" reduced impact, and several alternative warnings were more effective than the existing alcohol warning label. Again warnings with the words "poison," "cancer," or "health problems" were the most powerful.

Experimental Effects of an Alcohol Warning Poster

Kalsher and colleagues[93] conducted a randomized field experiment of an alcohol facts poster at several college fraternities. The posters were strategically placed in high traffic areas such as meeting rooms, bulletin boards, kitchens, and bathrooms. In Experiment 1, 134 undergraduate and graduate students at eight social fraternities were assigned randomly to each of four conditions in a Solomon four-group design:

1. Pretest–posttest without an intervention;
2. Pretest intervention posttest;
3. Intervention then posttest; and
4. Posttest without an intervention.

The poster significantly increased knowledge of alcohol-related information in an individual-level statistical analysis. In a replication experiment with a new poster that included less well-known risks of alcohol use and only one fraternity in each of the four conditions, student knowledge of the risks of alcohol written on the poster again improved significantly. The researchers reported some evidence that heavier drinkers may have reduced their alcohol consumption in the intervention groups. Similar effects were observed in a sample of college-age females.[94]

Summary of Deliberate Studies

The noticeability or conspicuousness of alcohol warnings is improved with horizontal placement, pictorials, color, and icons. Borders do not appear to have a substantial effect. Combined video and audio presentation of warnings leads to more substantial memory for television advertisements with warnings. There is evidence that persons read the alcohol warning label because recognition memory is positively associated with alcohol use—a measure of repeated exposure to the warning. Warnings that include words such as poison, cancer, or health problems appear to elicit avoidance responses, but the effects of adding these words to the existing label needs to be explored further.

A methodological explanation of Snyder and Blood's conclusion that warnings may make alcohol more attractive to male alcohol users is the confounding of gender and drinking status. Because there were no male nondrinkers included in the analysis, the differences may be owing to gender rather than the experimental manipulation. A substantive explanation comes from the theory of cognitive dissonance. When persons who drink alcohol are confronted with negative information about drinking, this creates an uncomfortable state of dissonance because of the inconsistency between the information and their own behavior. The drinkers perceive more benefits and fewer risks to make their beliefs consistent with their behavior.

Malouff et al.'s study suggested that a prompt to the warning decreases consumption and that increased memory for the warnings leads to less drinking. Because no intervention was delivered to control subjects, an alternative explanation is that contact with the experimenter reduced alcohol use. The study would have been improved with a control group of persons who were asked if they could remember the alcohol percentage of their last drink or whether there is a warning on cigarets. It is possible that heavier drinkers, who also have more accurate memory for the warning, are most sensitive to a stranger commenting on their drinking.

The effects of alcohol warnings will be clarified with more studies that combine field settings and randomization to experimental conditions.[93,94] Kalsher et al.'s results would be more convincing if enough fraternities were included so that the unit of analysis matched the unit of assignment. Kalsher and colleagues mentioned valuable future experiments with this design, including variations of poster format and test of effects on alcohol use and alcohol problems.

In deliberate studies, the experimental control of exposure to warnings increases the validity of the research conclusions. But deliberate studies typically artificially reproduce the conditions under which the real effects of the label may operate. In particular, many laboratory studies include one or a few exposures to warnings, which is unlike the repeated exposure to various[95] warnings that actually occurs. With the exception of the work of Laughery and colleagues, laboratory studies have focused on college students, so the results may not be generalizable to other populations.

Natural Experiments

Natural experiments provide ecologically valid evaluation of the warning label but experimental control of important factors is lacking. It was not possible, for example, to randomly assign states to either receive beverage containers with or without warning labels. The natural experiments have consisted of survey studies with measures taken both before and after the label was introduced. The effects of the warning label have been studied with interviews of pregnant women, telephone surveys of adults, and questionnaires completed by adults and adolescents. The variables measured are shown in Table 2. Studies are organized by the sample studied.

National Phone Survey of Adults

There is considerable public support for a warning label on alcoholic beverages. A Gallup survey of US adults ($N = 1559$), during October 1986, found 79% of respondents favored a federal law requiring warnings on alcoholic beverages.[96] A national survey of adults, taken June–July 1989, before the warning label appeared ($N = 2006$), found even higher public support (87%).[97] Warning labels were second in support to educational programs and were supported more than many other measures, including server interventions and treatment. Support was high even though 89% did not believe that the warnings would have much effect on heavy drinkers and 69% thought that people already knew the hazards associated with drinking. A large number of respondents, 84%, felt that labels should be put on alcoholic beverages even if there is only the slightest suspicion of danger, and 60% felt that the warnings would be an effective way to change people's behavior.

In a cross-sectional follow-up survey ($N = 2017$) during June, July, and August 1991, support for the warning label increased from 87–91% from the prelabel measurement and was then the most highly supported of 13 alcohol control policies.[25] Even if the one-third of the sample who did not participate in the survey were not in favor of alcohol warnings, the majority of all persons would favor them. As Kaskutas pointed out, the public may favor warnings because they are less restrictive than other alcohol control policies and the current norm is less tolerant of alcohol abuse.

Using the same sample just described,[61,98] Kaskutas and Greenfield[99,100] found an increase from 8–27% (21% adjusted for false positives) in the percentage of persons who reported seeing the warning. There was no statistically significant increase in knowledge of the health risks on the label, but the knowledge of these messages was already very high. There were no positive changes in self-reported behaviors related to the hazards mentioned

Table 2
Measures Used in Alcohol Warning Natural Experiments

Study	Support	Awareness	Exposure	Beliefs	Risk perceptions	Memory	Alcohol use	Risky behavior
Fenaughty and MacKinnon (1993)[118]		X	X	X		X		
Graves (1993)[101]		X		X	X	X	X	X
Greenfield and Kaskutas (1993)[61]		X	X		X	X	X	X
Hankin et al. (1993)[56]		X						
Hankin et al. (1993)[109]								
Hankin et al. (1993)[110]							X	
Hilton and Kaskutas (1991)[97]	X							
Kaskutas (1993)[25]	X							
Kaskutas and Greenfield (1992)[100]		X	X		X			
MacKinnon et al. (1993)[58,116]		X	X	X		X	X	
Mayer et al. (1991)[103]		X	X		X	X	X	
Marin (1990)[114]		X						
Marin (1994)[115]		X						
Mazis et al. (1991)[102]		X	X		X	X		
Scammon et al. (1991)[59]		X			X	X	X	
Scammon et al. (1992)[104]		X	X		X	X		

on the warning. Drinkers and young persons were more likely to have seen the label. Compared to persons who had not seen the label, persons who had seen the label were more knowledgeable about the risks, reported higher levels of driving after drinking, said they limited their drinking because of driving, and had more conversations about drinking and driving and the risk of drinking while pregnant.

Graves[101] used the same data from US adults but included surveys in 1990 and 1991 from residents in Ontario, Canada ($N = 1045$ and 1028, respectively) where a warning label is not required. US respondents ($N = 2000$ and 2006, respectively) were more aware of the label (35% in 1991) and were more likely to say that risks both on and off the label were more likely to appear on the warning label than Ontario respondents. The majority of Ontario and US respondents believed the risks mentioned on the warning label. US respondents were more likely to believe that pregnant women should not drink, and that drinking may cause health problems. Differences between Ontario and US respondents may be caused by the alcohol warning label, but there are many other variables that may explain these differences, e.g., legislative activity and sample differences.

As noted by Graves, a more rigorous test of the alcohol warning label is the test for different trends in the Ontario vs the US sample. Only 4 of the 21 tests (21 dependent variables are presented in the tables) of different trends were statistically significant. Three of these effects suggest more positive trends for Ontario than for US respondents—awareness of the operating machinery risk, danger of any alcohol use while pregnant, and the danger of driving after five or more drinks increased. The positive effect for US respondents was the increase in the percent of persons who did not drive after drinking.

Gallup Telephone Survey of Adults

Six questions were asked as part of the monthly Gallup organization survey in May 1989 ($N = 1008$) and 1990 ($N = 1020$).[102] Approximately one-third of working telephone numbers provided interviews for the study. In the responding sample, there was a significant increase in persons responding that alcohol beverages were "very harmful" after the label appeared compared to before the label appeared. In May 1989, 23.3% of the respondents reported that it is very likely that alcohol beverages have warnings compared to 35.1% in May 1990. Alcohol users were also more likely to report that alcohol was very harmful after the label appeared. Younger persons were more likely to say that there was a warning label. In 1989, 2.9% of the sample responded that the warning label was very likely to contain the birth defects message and in 1990 11% noted that this risk was on the warning label. Alcohol drinkers and middle income respondents appeared to have the largest increase in this belief.

Survey of Mormon and Non-Mormon Utah Residents

Mayer and colleagues[103,104] evaluated the effects of the alcohol warning label by taking advantage of a special characteristic of Utah to create a nonequivalent, nonexposed, comparison group of Mormon respondents. Many Utah residents are Mormons who not only abstain from alcohol consumption but also are unlikely to come into contact with the warning on beverages because the state of Utah sells alcohol beverages, other than beer with a low percentage alcohol, in special state-owned liquor stores.

Data were collected during April, July, and October 1989, before the warning was required to appear, and January, April, and July 1990 (minimum $N = 400$ each month), after the label was required to appear from Mormon and non-Mormon Utah residents. Measures were perceptions of alcohol-related risks not on the label (cirrhosis of the liver and leukemia), perceptions of risk on the label (drinking when driving and drinking when pregnant), knowledge and awareness of the warning label and the Utah warning poster, and monthly alcohol use. Gender, age, and region were comparable with 1980 census data for Utah. Overall, Mormons were less aware of the label and the poster and attributed greater risks to alcohol use.

Followup data were collected from October 1990, January 1991, and April 1991.[104] Awareness of the warning label increased substantially among non-Mormons and less devout Mormons in comparison to devout Mormons. Increases in awareness were largest among alcohol users. Recall was higher for the two risks mentioned on the warning label (drinking and driving and birth defects) and lower for the risks not mentioned in the warning (leukemia and liver cirrhosis). Across the six followup waves, 39.4% of respondents correctly identified that the two risks on the label were actually on the label and the two risks not on the label were not on the label.

Survey of Pregnant Black Women

Hankin and colleagues[105–113] studied the effects of the alcohol warning label among pregnant Black women at an inner city Detroit prenatal clinic. They found increases in awareness from 35% before November 18, 1989 to 37% from November 18, 1989–May 31, 1990, and to 56% from June 1–September 30, 1991 ($N = 5169$). There was some evidence that the awareness of the warning label did not increase until March 1990.[109] There was no evidence of a change in consumption either while pregnant or 2 wk before their first prenatal visit.

In a subsequent study ($N = 4397$), the researchers found a statistically significant decline in alcohol consumption during pregnancy of .0065 ounces per day among nonrisk drinkers but not among risk drinkers (.0037 ounces per day) from June 1–September 30, 1991.[56] Risk drinkers were defined as persons who drank .5 ounces or more alcohol per day.[108,109]

Survey of Hispanic and Non-Hispanic Adults in San Francisco

Marin[114,115] conducted two studies of San Francisco residents in predominantly Hispanic areas. A total of 644 persons were interviewed by telephone during June, July, and August 1989, and 1 yr later, 369 of the respondents were interviewed again. Respondents answered questions in their language of choice. Males, younger persons, and persons with less education were less likely to be interviewed the second time.

Awareness was the percentage of respondents who said they saw, read, or heard about the message. As a result, the percentages are much higher than in other studies with slight increases in awareness of the birth defects (57.2–59.7%) and impaired driving (41.1–48.8%) messages. There was also an increase in awareness of the risk of smoking to the fetus, suggesting that the alcohol risk changes may be attributable to secular trends. More acculturated persons had a larger increase in awareness of messages than the less acculturated persons.

The second survey was cross-sectional[115] with data collected from 1204 Hispanic and 536 non-Hispanic Whites in 1990 and 1569 Hispanics and 520 non-Hispanic White persons in 1991. There were changes in awareness of the existence of a warning for beer and wine. There was also a small increase for the cigarette warning making the changes in beer and wine difficult to attribute the alcohol warning label. Marin suggested that Spanish versions of signs and warning posters may lead to larger increases in awareness among Hispanics.

Survey of Marion County, Indiana Adolescents

Awareness of the alcohol labeling law and exposure to, beliefs about, and memory for the government-mandated alcohol warning label were measured in a sample of adolescents immediately before the label was required to appear (in the fall of 1989) and for the 2 yr after the label was required ($N = 1211$, 2006, and 3174 for 12th graders and $N = 2295$, 3625, and 3867 for 10th graders).[58,116] For 12th graders over the 3-yr period, there were substantial increases in awareness of the alcohol warning label law (19, 43, and 48%), but not the cigaret warning label law. Reported exposure to warning increased (26, 41, 47%) as did memory for the warning label

(3.6, 4.3, and 4.5 correct on a scale of 0–6). There were small changes in beliefs about the risks written on the label and a slight decrease in reported alcohol use. Effects for 10th graders led to identical conclusions. In both grades, the correlation between alcohol use and recognition memory for the alcohol warnings was not significant in the prelabel measurement but is statistically significant in postlabel measurements. If the warning label was not read, then the correlation between alcohol use and memory should be zero for all measurements.

Effects of the New York and Arizona Alcohol Warning Poster

In a study of the New York City Warning Poster, 54% of the persons interviewed before the warning poster appeared mentioned birth defects as a possible consequence of a pregnant woman's alcohol consumption. A year later, after the poster had appeared, 68% mentioned birth defects.[117] The results of this study suggest that warning posters do have the capability of increasing awareness of the possible consequences of a pregnant woman's alcohol consumption.

There is evidence that the appearance of the Arizona warning poster led to increased awareness of, exposure to, and memory for the warning poster[118] in a sample of college students measured before ($N = 362$) and after ($N = 332$) the legislation became effective on January 1, 1992. The appearance of the warning poster was associated with greater exposure, awareness, and memory. There was inconsistent evidence regarding the association between the appearance of the warning poster and beliefs. Secular trends did not appear to be responsible for these changes. The effects were maintained 6 and 12 mo after the poster appeared.[116]

Summary of Effects of Natural Experiments

With the possible exception of the longitudinal study of San Francisco Hispanics, the results of the natural experiments on the alcohol warning label are consistent. Overall, the studies suggest effects in the early stages of behavior change.[55] The results are consistent across two national telephone surveys of adults;[98,102] surveys of Marion County, Indiana adolescents;[58] interviews of pregnant women in a Detroit hospital;[56] and interviews with Utah adults.[59] The effects of the warning poster show a similar pattern.[118] There are substantial changes in awareness of and exposure to the warning. Persons also appear to be reading the warning because memory for its content has increased.

In contrast to effects on awareness and memory, there has not been much evidence that beliefs about or perceptions of the risks of alcohol use have

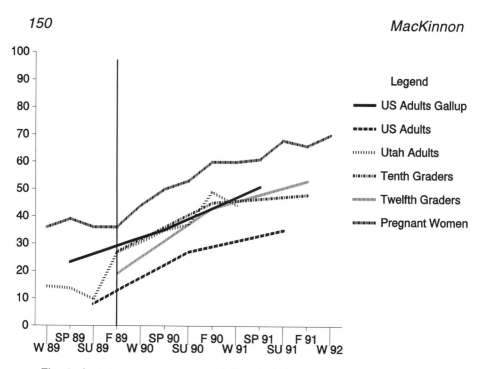

Fig. 1. Awareness percentages of the alcohol warning label. Awareness was measured differently across the samples: US adults Gallop,[102] US adults,[97] Utah adults,[103] 10th graders,[58] 12th graders,[58] and pregnant women.[109]

changed in the 2 yr after the label appeared. One explanation is that there is a ceiling effect on these beliefs because approx 90% of respondents already believe these risks. Mazis et al.,[102] however, found an increase in the perceived harm of alcohol use with a measure that did not have a ceiling effect.

Convincing evidence for effects on behaviors is not yet available because, in part, few studies have evaluated effects on these variables. Hankin and colleagues did find a reduction in drinking among gravidas, but only among low-risk, not high-risk, drinkers. Across studies there has not been evidence that alcohol use has decreased. Nor has there been evidence for declines in driving after drinking, drinking while pregnant, drinking while operating machinery, or health problems that can be attributed to the warning label.

Hilton[57] suggested that effects of the alcohol warning on behavior may not occur until the percentage of persons who are aware of the alcohol label is similar to the percentage aware of the cigaret label, or about 90%. The awareness percentages across the available studies is shown in Fig. 1. The average linear regression line across studies predicts 90% awareness of the alcohol warning label in the spring of 1994. According to

Hilton's prediction, warning effects on alcohol problems may be present when data from the spring of 1994 becomes available.

Methodological Issues

In each of the telephone surveys, over one-third of potential respondents did not participate in the survey. The data were weighted for age, sex, number of eligible adults contacted, and telephone numbers per household. It is likely, however, that the missing subjects may lead to some bias in the cross-sectional results but missing data are an unlikely explanation of the changes over the measurements. The changes over time may be biased if the tendency to answer telephone surveys or the sample studied changed over time. Other problems with telephone surveys are the number of homes without telephones and the often unknown characteristics of persons who refuse to complete the survey.[119] Similar criticisms can be made about the interview data in Utah[104] and Detroit[56] and the questionnaire data from adolescents.[58] It is very important, therefore, that results are replicated across samples and data collection methods.

The use of pre- as well as postlabel measures is especially important because respondents in all studies indicated that they had seen the warning label before it was required to appear. There are several explanations of this including the presence of warning labels on containers prior to the legislation and similar warnings on television, radio, and other sources. Another explanation is the phenomenon of acquiescence bias where subjects tend to answer in the affirmative to please the interviewer.[109,120] It is likely that acquiescence bias may operate for other measures besides exposure to the warning. Therefore, it is important to include measures taken prior to the legal requirement of warnings and comparison measures such as distractor risks in memory measures.

The most common design used to evaluate the alcohol warning label is the one group prelabel, postlabel design. The difference between pre- and postlabel measures is the estimate of effect of the warning label. Alternative explanations of changes in warning label measures from the pre- to the postlabel measurement are history, statistical regression, maturation, and testing and instrumentation.[121]

The maturation, repeated testing, instrument change, or statistical regression alternative explanations are not likely to explain changes because most studies obtained random samples from the same age range, measured variables the same way, and did not measure the same subjects before and after the label appeared. The study of Hispanics[115] obtained data from the same subjects at two time points so aging or maturation may explain effects in this study.

History is an explanation of observed effects if there are other historical events that explain changes rather than the introduction of the label. Perhaps the best example of this alternative explanation is for the risk of birth defects warning. Many other campaigns to increase awareness of the risk of drinking while pregnant are in progress including warning posters in certain states, and media and medical campaigns. Any changes in awareness of this risk may be owing to these other activities rather than the warning label.

To reduce the history alternative explanation of any observed changes in warning label measures, researchers have used comparison groups. Mayer and colleagues[59] obtained label effects among non-Mormons but not in a sample of Mormons who are less likely to be exposed to alcohol and the warning label than non-Mormons. Graves[101] used respondents in Ontario, Canada as a group relatively unexposed to the US alcohol warnings, although differences between the US and Canada were complicated because no prelabel measure of Ontario residents was available. Thus differences between the two locations are difficult to attribute to the label. Increases over time in the US, but not Ontario, residents suggests that these changes could be owing to the label. Unfortunately, there was not extensive evidence that the changes in the US sample were greater than in the Ontario sample. Trends in future data collection should clarify the effects of the label.

Another more common procedure to address alternative explanations of effects are comparison variables that should not be affected by the alcohol warning label, but would be affected by response biases' or general trends in perceptions of warnings.[59] MacKinnon et al.,[58] for example, found that awareness of the cigaret warning label did not change, while awareness of the alcohol warning label increased substantially. Several researchers found improved memory for alcohol risks on the warning label but not for risks not on the warning label.[58,104]

The statistical conclusion validity of the research studies have been generally sufficient with most studies having adequate statistical power. A possible exception are some subgroup analyses. Relatively robust categorical and descriptive analysis methods have been used. Researchers have been cautious about accepting the null hypothesis, although mass media and some researchers have attributed lack of significant effects to failure of the warning. The reliability of treatment implementation may be problematic as there is evidence that the label was placed on some alcoholic beverages before the November 1989 legal requirement which may dilute estimates of warning label effects. Alternatively, warning labels did not appear on all beverages until well after November 1989 because alcohol containers on the shelf before November 1989 did not require labels.

Discussion and Future Directions

The natural experiments provide evidence that persons are aware of the label and have seen it.[58,59,61,102,109] In laboratory experiments, subjects exposed to warnings are more likely to report seeing them.[28,89,90] Subjects exposed to the warnings also appear to process the warning label to the extent that their memory for the warning is enhanced. The effect on memory has been observed in several field studies[58,59] and laboratory exposure to the warnings is associated with the improved, but not perfect, memory for the warning.[77,85,89,90]

Amount of alcohol use is associated with memory for the content of the label[58,77] and the effects of the warning label appear to be stronger among alcohol users.[102] An explanation for this effect is that alcohol use is a proxy measure for exposure to the warning. Since alcohol use is associated with repeated exposure to the warning, this increases the likelihood of processing of the content of the label. It could also be predicted that the relationship between alcohol use and memory for the warnings should be negative because understanding the message in the warning should decrease consumption. It appears at this stage in the effect of the warning label, the exposure effect is much stronger than any deterrent effect of warnings. The correlation between alcohol use and memory is not large (.1–.3), perhaps in part due to this deterrent effect. Malouff et al.'s study of Florida bar patrons is consistent with the deterrent effect as they found a negative correlation between alcohol consumed and memory for the warning. The negative correlation could be owing to stronger cuing effects for persons who drink more, and drinkers have better memory for the warning owing to exposure. Experimental and longitudinal studies of alcohol consumption and related problems and memory for the warning label are necessary to disentangle these effects.

In both the deliberate and natural experiments there is not much evidence for an effect of alcohol warnings on perception of the risks of alcohol use perhaps because most people already know these risks. However, perceptions of these risks have not decreased substantially suggesting that overwarning or the false alarm effects mentioned earlier may not be operating. An important future research question is whether increased perception of the risk of using alcohol is necessary to observe effects on behavior.

There is not much evidence that the warning label has actually affected behavior. Hankin et al.[109] found that, in pregnant women, alcohol consumption among low-risk drinkers declined but not among high-risk drinkers after the label appeared. Malouff et al.'s study suggests that cues to the warning may reduce alcohol use. Other studies have found nonsignificant declines in alcohol use.[58] Kaskutas[122] found that 55% of respondents said the label had affected their drinking. The field studies, if continued, will provide ecologically valid information on the effects of the warning as exposure to the label reaches a level that may change behavior. Future research should focus on these potential long-term effects of the label on problem behaviors. Comprehensive models for the relations among awareness, risk perception, memory, and behaviors should increase understanding of the effects of alcohol warnings.[29] In particular, it would be helpful to use data from warning label studies to test McGuire's communication model, and to see if the warning label functions as a cue in the health belief model[61] or the expectancy-accessibility model.[29] The extent to which other communication or health data fit these models would also provide insight into the potential effects of the alcohol warning label.

There are sources of data on alcohol problems available in the national archives such as the National Center for Health Statistics that may be useful to test effects of the warning label. Often these data sets include measures both before and after the warning label was introduced. It may be possible to study changes in the incidence of behaviors mentioned on the label such as traffic fatalities and FAS. Control variables or nonequivalent groups such as similar data from Canada[101] should prove useful in further evaluations of the label.

Laboratory studies combining methods from several studies, such as manipulation of warnings suggested by avoidance responses with experimental procedures used by Snyder and Blood[28] and Laughery et al.,[82] may be informative. Snyder and Blood's findings that warnings increase the perceived benefits of alcohol deserves replication. Kalsher et al.'s[93] randomized field study on the effects of posters provides a model for field experiments.

It remains to be determined if combining the warning label with other alcohol prevention strategies can change alcohol use. Combining multiple exposures or cues to such interventions may lead to more substantial effects on behavior.[95] The extent to which the warning label contributes to a societal norm less tolerant to alcohol use should be examined. The effects of proposed advertisement warnings will provide an opportunity to test repeated exposures to warning label messages if the law is passed.

Future research should address the potential negative effects of the alcohol warning label such as overwarning and the false alarm effect. Studies of message repetition on persuasion may increase understanding of repeated exposure to the warning label. These studies may be improved with stronger links with the research literature on risk perception[123,124] and media health campaigns.[125,126]

Alcohol warnings have considerable public support and represent a large scale communication intervention. The research conducted during the first 3 yr of the warning label has shed light on its effects. We already know much more about the effects of the alcohol label than the cigaret label. The effect of warnings on alcohol use and alcohol-related problems remains to be determined.

Acknowledgments

The chapter was supported by Grant AA8547 from the National Institute on Alcohol Abuse and Alcoholism. I thank Alan Stacy, Lee Kaskutas, Mike Hilton, Liva Nohre, and Mary Ann Pentz for comments on this chapter.

References

[1]H. Haggard, ed. (1945) Editorial: the proposed Massachusetts "label" and its place in education against inebriety. *Q. J. Stud. Alcohol* **6,** 1–3.

[2]Alcoholic Beverage Labeling Act of 1988, H.R. 5409, Public Law No. 100-690.

[3]US Department of Health and Human Services (1986) *Toward a National Plan to Combat Alcohol Abuse and Alcoholism.* A report to the United States Congress. National Institute on Alcohol Abuse and Alcoholism, Rockville, MD.

[4]US Department of Health and Human Services (1988) *Surgeon General's Workshop on Drunk Driving.* Author, Rockville, MD.

[5]E. L. Abel and R. J. Sokol (1991) A revised estimate of the economic impact of fetal alcohol syndrome. *Recent Dev. Alcohol* **9,** 117–126.

[6]US Department of Health and Human Services (1989) *Research on Economic and Socioeconomic Issues in the Prevention, Treatment, and Epidemiology of Alcohol Abuse and Alcoholism.* Request for Applications. National Institute on Alcohol Abuse and Alcoholism, Rockville, MD.

[7]P. J. Gruenewald (1993) Alcohol problems and the control of availability: theoretical and empirical issues, in *Economics and the Prevention of Alcohol Related Problems.* Research monograph 25. National Institute on Alcohol Abuse and Alcoholism, US Department of Health and Human Services, Rockville, MD, pp. 59–90.

[8]M. Grossman, D. Coate, and G. M. Arluck (1987) Price sensitivity of alcoholic beverages in the United States, in *Control Issues in Alcohol Abuse Prevention: Strategies for States and Communities.* H. D. Holder, ed. JAI, Greenwich, CT, pp. 169–198.

[9]P. Cook and G. Tauchen (1982) The effect of liquor taxes on heavy drinking. *Bell J. Econ.* **13,** 379–390.

[10]A. C. Wagenaar (1983) *Alcohol, Young Drivers, and Traffic Accidents: Effects of Minimum-Age Laws.* Heath, Lexington, MA.

[11]D. Coate and M. Grossman (1988) Effects of alcoholic beverage prices and legal drinking ages on youth alcohol use. *J. Law Econ.* **31,** 145–171.

[12]P. M. O'Malley and A. C. Wagenaar (1991) Effects of minimum drinking age laws on alcohol use, related behaviors and traffic crash involvement among American youth: 1976–1987. *J. Stud. Alcohol* **52,** 478–491.

[13]US Department of Health and Human Services (1993) *Eighth Special Report to the U.S. Congress on Alcohol and Health.* Author, Rockville, MD.

[14]L. Evans (1991) *Traffic Safety and the Driver.* Reinhold, New York.

[15]H. L. Ross (1984) Social control through deterrence: drinking-and-driving laws. *Annu. Rev. Soc.* **10,** 21–35.

[16]G. J. Botvin, E. Baker, L. Dusenburg, S. Tortu, and E. M. Botvin (1990) Preventing adolescent drug abuse through multimodal cognitive behavioral approach: results of a 3-year study. *J. Consult. Clin. Psychol.* **58,** 437–446.

[17]W. B. Hansen (1992) A review of school-based drug prevention: a review of the state of the art in curriculum, 1980–1990. *Health Educ. Res.* **7,** 403–430.

[18]M. A. Pentz, J. H. Dwyer, D. P. MacKinnon, B. R. Flay, W. B. Hansen, E. Wang, and C. A. Johnson (1989) A multi-community trial for primary prevention of adolescent drug abuse: effects on drug use prevalence. *JAMA* **261,** 3259–3266.

[19]C. K. Atkin (1990) Effects of televised alcohol messages on teenage drinking patterns. *J. Adolesc. Health Care* **11,** 10–24.

[20]M. R. Robberson and R. W. Rogers (1988) Beyond fear appeals: negative and positive persuasive appeals to health and self-esteem. *J. Appl. Soc. Psychol.* **18,** 277–287.

[21]R. G. Smart (1988) Does alcohol advertising affect overall consumption? A review of empirical studies. *J. Stud. Alcohol* **49,** 314–323.

[22]P. P. Aitken, D. R. Eadie, D. S. Leathar, R. E. McNeill, and A. C. Scott (1988) Television advertisements for alcoholic drinks do reinforce under-age drinking. *Br. J. Addict.* **83,** 1399–1419.

[23]G. Gerbner, L. Gross, M. Morgan, and N. Signorielli (1986) Living with television: the dynamics of the cultivation process, in *Perspectives on Media Effects.* J. Bryant and D. Zillmann, eds. Erlbaum, Hillsdale, NJ, pp. 17–40.

[24]B. R. Flay (1986) Mass media linkages with school-based programs for drug abuse prevention. *J. School Health* **56,** 402–406.

[25]L. A. Kaskutas (1993) Changes in public attitudes toward alcohol control policies since the warning label mandate of 1988. *J. Public Policy Marketing* **12,** 30–37.

[26]S. G. Hadden (1986) *Read the Label: Reducing the Risk by Providing Information.* Westview, Boulder, CO.

[27]M. R. Lehto and J. M. Miller (1986) *Warnings. Volume I: Fundamentals, Design, and Evaluation Methodologies.* Fuller Technical Publications, Ann Arbor, MI.

[28]L. B. Snyder and D. J. Blood (1992) Caution: alcohol advertising and the Surgeon General's alcohol warnings may have adverse effects on young adults. *J. Appl. Commun. Res.* **20,** 37–53.

[29]A. W. Stacy, D. P. MacKinnon, and M. A. Pentz (1993) Generality and specificity in health behavior: application to warning-label and social influence expectancies. *J. Appl. Psychol.* **78,** 611–627.

[30]G. A. Peters (1991) Warnings, notices, and safety information, in *Sourcebook on Asbestos Diseases, Vol. 5, Asbestos Abatement.* G. A. Peters and B. J. Peters, eds. Butterworth, Salem, NH, pp. 695–805.

[31]M. R. Lehto and J. M. Miller (1988) The effectiveness of warning labels. *J. Prod. Liability* **11,** 225–270.

[32]R. L. McCarthy, J. P. Finnegan, S. Krumm-Scott, and G. E. McCarthy (1984) Product information presentation, user behavior, and safety, in *Proceedings of the Human Factors Society 28th Annual Meeting.* Human Factors Society, Santa Monica, CA, pp. 81–85.

[33]M. S. Wogalter, S. S. Godfrey, G. A. Fontenelle, D. R. Desaulniers, P. R. Rothestein, and K. R. Laughery (1987) Effectiveness of warnings, in *Proceedings of the Human Factors Society 31st Annual Meeting.* Human Factors Society, Santa Monica, CA, pp. 599–612.

[34]R. C. Engs (1989) Do warning labels on alcoholic beverages deter alcohol abuse? *J. School Health* **59,** 116–118.

[35]A. H. Lipson and W. S. Webster (1990) Response to letters dealing with warning labels on alcoholic beverages (letter to the editor). *Teratology* **41,** 479–481.

[36]R. E. Seegmiller, J. C. Carey, and R. M. Fineman (1990) Reply to: response to letters dealing with warning labels on alcoholic beverages (letter to the editor). *Teratoloay* **41,** 483–484.

[37]J. R. West (1990) Reply to: response to letters dealing with warning labels on alcoholic beverages (letter to the editor). *Teratology* **41,** 485–487.

[38]C. C. Willhite and S. A. Book (1990) Reply to: response to letters dealing with warning labels on alcoholic beverages (letter to the editor). *Teratology* **41,** 489.

[39]R. N. Mayer and D. L. Scammon (1992) Caution: weak product warnings may be hazardous to corporate health. *J. Bus. Res.* **24,** 347–359.

[40]S. M. Andreas (1988) A case for alcohol beverage warning labels: duty to warn of dangers of consumption (Hon v. Stroh Brewery Co.). *Missouri Law Rev.* **53,** 555–565.

[41]C. H. Dukes (1989) Alcohol manufacturers and the duty to warn: an analysis of recent case law in light of the alcoholic beverage labeling act of 1988. *Emory Law J.* **38,** 1189–1222.

[42]C. E. Khoury (1989) Warning labels may be hazardous to your health: common-law and statutory responses to alcoholic beverage manufacturers' duty to warn. *Cornell Law Rev.* **75,** 158–189.

[43]V. E. Schwartz and R. W. Driver (1983) Warnings in the workplace: the need for a synthesis of law and communication theory. *Univ. Cincinnati Law Rev.* **52,** 38–83.

[44]M. Ursic (1985) Product safety warnings: a legal review. *J. Public Policy Marketing* **4,** 80–90.

[45]R. W. Driver (1987) A communication model for determining the appropriateness of on-product warnings. *IEEE Trans. Prof. Commun.* **30,** 157–163.

[46]A. S. Weinstein, A. D. Twerski, H. R. Piehler, and W. A. Donaher (1978) Warnings and disclaimers, in *Products Liability and the Reasonably Safe Product: A Guide for Management, Design and Marketing.* Wiley, New York, pp. 60–74.

[47]A. D. Twerski, A. S. Weinstein, W. A. Donaher, and H. R. Piehler (1976) The use and abuse of warnings in products liability: design defect litigation comes of age. *Cornell Law Rev.* **4,** 495–540.

[48]B. H. Kantowitz and R. D. Sorkin (1983) *Human Factors: Understanding People–System Relationships.* Wiley, New York.

[49]J. T. Cacioppo and R. E. Petty (1979) Effects of message repetition on argument processing, recall, and persuasion. *J. Pers. Soc. Psychol.* **37,** 97–109.

[50]J. T. Cacioppo and R. E. Petty (1989) Effects of message repetition on argument processing, recall, and persuasion. *Basic Appl. Soc. Psychol.* **10,** 3–12.

[51]D. P. MacKinnon, A. Bryan, and A. Barr (1993) *Four Studies on the Effects of Multiple Warnings: Overwarning and the False Alarm Effect.* Project ABLE technical report, Tempe, AZ.

[52]S. Breznitz (1984) *Cry Wolf: The Psychology of False Alarms.* Erlbaum, Hillsdale, NJ.

[53]G. M. Goldhaber and M. A. deTurck (1988) Effects of consumers' familiarity with a product on attention to and compliance with warnings. *J. Products Liability* **11,** 29–37.

[54]K. R. Laughery and J. W. Brelsford (1991) Receiver characteristics in safety communications, in *Proceedings of the Human Factors Society 35th Annual Meeting*. Human Factors Society, Santa Monica, CA, pp. 1068–1072.

[55]W. J. McGuire (1980) The communication-persuasion model and health-risk labeling, in *Banbury Report: Product Labeling and Health Risks*. L. A. Morris, M. B. Mazis, and I. Barofsky, eds. Cold Spring Harbor Laboratory, Cold Spring Harbor, NY, pp. 99–122.

[56]J. Hankin, I. Firestone, J. Sloan, J. Ager, A. Goodman, R. Sokol, and S. Martier (1993) The impact of the alcohol warning label on drinking during pregnancy. *J. Public Policy Marketing* **12,** 10–18.

[57]M. E. Hilton (1993) An overview of recent findings on alcoholic beverage warning labels. *J. Public Policy Marketing* **12,** 1–9.

[58]D. P. MacKinnon, M. A. Pentz, and A. W. Stacy (1993) The alcohol warning label and adolescents: the first year. *Am. J. Public Health* **83,** 585–587.

[59]D. L. Scammon, R. N. Mayer, and K. R. Smith (1991) Alcohol warnings: how do you know when you have had one too many? *J. Public Policy Marketing* **10,** 214–228.

[60]N. K. Janz and M. H. Becker (1984) The health belief model: a decade later. *Health Educ. Q.* **11,** 1–47.

[61]T. K. Greenfield and L. A. Kaskutas (1993) Early impacts of alcoholic beverage warning labels: national study findings relevant to drinking and driving behavior. *Safety Sci.* **16,** 689–707.

[62]A. W. Stacy, M. Krank, and G. A. Marlatt (1989) *Expectancy Effects on Alcohol Use: A Critical and Integrative Theoretical Review*. Unpublished manuscript (available from A. Stacy, USC, 35 N. Lake Ave, Suite 200, Pasadena, CA 91101, or Alan Marlatt, Dept. of Psych, NI-25, UW, Seattle, WA 98195).

[63]A. W. Stacy and K. F. Widaman (1987) *A Positivity Bias in Attitude Models of Alcohol Use*. Paper presented at the meeting of the American Psychological Association, August, New York, NY.

[64]R. S. Wyer and J. Hartwick (1984) The recall and use of belief statements as bases for judgments: some determinants and implications. *J. Exp. Soc. Psychol.* **20,** 65–85.

[65]L. Nohre, D. MacKinnon, and A. Stacy (1993) *Controlled Associations of Alcohol Use Consequences*. Poster presented at the Western Psychological Association Annual Meeting, Phoenix, AZ.

[66]J. D. Leckenby and J. T. Plummer (1983) Advertising stimulus measurement and assessment research: a review of advertising testing methods. *Curr. Issues Res. Advertising* **2,** 135–165.

[67]US Department of Health and Human Services, Public Health Service (1964) *Smoking and Health*. Report of the Advisory Committee to the Surgeon General of the Public Health Service. DHEW Pub. No. (PHS) 1103. Govt. Printing Office, Washington, DC.

[68]K. E. Warner (1981) Cigarette smoking in the 1970's: the impact of the anti-smoking campaign on consumption. *Science* **211,** 729–731.

[69]K. E. Warner and H. A. Murt (1983) Premature deaths avoided by the antismoking campaign. *Am. J. Public Health* **73,** 645–650.

[70]R. F. Beltramini (1988) Perceived believability of warning label information presented in cigarette advertising. *J. Advert.* **17,** 26–32.

[71]G. Bhalla and J. Lastovicka (1984) The impact of changing cigarette warning message content and format. *Adv. Consumer Res.* **11**, 305–310.

[72]B. Loken and B. Howard-Pitney (1988) Effectiveness of cigarette advertisements on women: an experimental study. *J. Appl. Psychol.* **73**, 378–382.

[73]R. M. Davis and J. S. Kendrick (1989) The Surgeon General's warnings in outdoor cigarette advertising: are they readable? *JAMA* **261**, 90–94.

[74]P. Fischer, J. Richards, E. Berman, and D. Krugman (1989) Recall and eye tracking study of adolescents viewing tobacco advertisements. *JAMA* **261**, 84–89.

[75]E. T. Popper and K. B. Murray (1989) Communication effectiveness and format effects on in-ad disclosure of health warnings. *J. Public Policy Marketing* **8**, 109–123.

[76]R. Brubaker and S. Mitby (1990) Health-risk warning labels on smokeless tobacco products: are they effective? *Addict. Behav.* **15**, 115–118.

[77]D. P. MacKinnon and A. M. Fenaughty (1993) Substance use and memory for health warning labels. *Health Psychol.* **12**, 147–150.

[78]P. Richardson, G. Reinhart, A. Rosenthal, C. Hayes, and R. Silver (1987) *Review of the Research Literature on the Effects of Health Warning Labels: A Report to the United States Congress*. National Institute of Alcohol Abuse and Alcoholism, Washington, DC.

[79]US Department of Health and Human Services (1990) *Seventh Special Report to the U.S. Congress on Alcohol and Health*. Author, Rockville, MD.

[80]R. Hingson, J. Howland, S. Morelock, and T. Heeren (1988) Legal interventions to reduce drunken driving and related fatalities among youthful drivers. *Alcohol, Drugs, Driving* **4**, 87–98.

[81]National Institute on Alcohol Abuse and Alcoholism (1989) *Program Announcement: Measuring the Impact of Alcohol Warning Labels*. Author, Rockville, MD (Request for applications AA-89-06 [Catalog of Domestic Assistance No. 13.273]).

[82]K. R. Laughery, S. L. Young, K. P. Vaubel, and J. W. Brelsford (1993) The noticeability of warnings on alcoholic beverage containers. *J. Public Policy Marketing* **12**, 38–56.

[83]S. S. Godfrey, K. R. Laughery, S. L. Young, K. P. Vaubel, J. W. Brelsford, K. A. Laughery, and E. Horn (1991) The new alcohol warning labels: how noticeable are they?, in *Proceedings of the Human Factors Society 35th Annual Meeting*. Human Factors Society, Santa Monica, CA, pp. 446–450.

[84]J. Malouff, N. Schutte, K. Wiener, C. Brancazio, and D. Fish (1993) Important characteristics of warning displays on alcohol containers. *J. Stud. Alcohol* **54**, 457–461.

[85]D. P. MacKinnon, A. W. Stacy, L. Nohre, and E. Geiselman (1992) Effects of processing depth on memory for the alcohol warning label, in *Proceedings of the Human Factors Society 35th Annual Meeting*. Human Factors Society, Santa Monica, CA, pp. 538–542.

[86]J. C. Andrews, R. G. Netemeyer, and S. Durvasula (1991) Believability and attitudes toward alcohol warning label information: the role of persuasive communications theory. *J. Public Policy Marketing* **9**, 1–15.

[87]J. C. Andrews, R. G. Netemeyer, and S. Durvasula (1991) Effects of consumption frequency on believability and attitudes toward alcohol warning labels. *J. Consumer Affairs* **25**, 323–338.

[88]J. C. Andrews, R. G. Netemeyer, and S. Durvasula (1993) The role of cognitive responses as mediators of alcohol warning label effects. *J. Public Policy Marketing* **12**, 57–68.

[89]S. J. Smith (1990) The impact of product usage warnings in alcoholic beverage advertising. *J. Public Policy Marketing* **9**, 16–29.

[90]T. Barlow and M. S. Wogalter (1993) Alcoholic beverage warnings in magazine and television advertisements. *J. Consumer Res.* **20**, 147–156.

[91]D. P. MacKinnon (1993) A choice-based method to compare alternative alcohol warning labels. *J. Stud. Alcohol* **54**, 614–617.

[92]D. P. MacKinnon, C. Nemeroff, and L. Nohre (1994) Avoidance responses to alcohol warning labels. *J. Appl. Soc. Psychol.* **24**, 733–753.

[93]M. J. Kalsher, S. W. Clarke, and M. S. Wogalter (1993) Communication of alcohol facts and hazards by a warning poster. *J. Public Policy Marketing* **12**, 78–90.

[94]M. J. Kalsher, M. S. Wogalter, and B. M. Racicot (1993) Development of posted alcohol warnings for specific target groups, in *Proceedings of the 1993 Marketing and Public Policy Conference.* M. J. Sheffet, ed. Michigan State University, Lansing, MI, pp. 133,134.

[95]L. A. Kaskutas and K. Graves (in press) Cumulative exposure to drinking-during-pregnancy health messages. *Am. J. Health Promotion.*

[96]The Gallup Report (1987) *Alcohol Use and Abuse in America.* Gallup Report No. 265, Princeton, NJ.

[97]M. E. Hilton and L. Kaskutas (1991) Public support for warning labels on alcoholic beverage containers. *Br. J. Addict.* **86**, 1323–1333.

[98]T. K. Greenfield, K. L. Graves, and L. A. Kaskutas (1993) Alcohol warning labels for prevention: national survey findings. *Alcohol Health Res. World* **17**, 67–75.

[99]L. A. Kaskutas and T. Greenfield (1991) Knowledge of warning labels on alcoholic beverage containers, in *Proceedings of the Human Factors Society 35th Annual Meeting.* Human Factors Society, Santa Monica, CA, pp. 441–445.

[100]L. A. Kaskutas and T. Greenfield (1992) First effects of warning labels on alcoholic beverage containers. *Drug Alcohol Depend.* **31**, 1–14.

[101]K. L. Graves (1993) An evaluation of the alcohol warning label: a comparison of the United States and Ontario, Canada in 1990 and 1991. *J. Public Pol. Marketing* **12**, 19–29.

[102]M. B. Mazis, L. A. Morris, and J. L. Swasy (1991) An evaluation of the alcohol warning label: initial survey results. *J. Public Policy Marketing* **10**, 229–241.

[103]R. N. Mayer, K. R. Smith, and D. L. Scammon (1991) Evaluating the impact of alcohol warning labels. *Adv. Consumer Res.* **18**, 706–714.

[104]D. L. Scammon, R. N. Mayer, and K. R. Smith (1992) The morning after: have consumers learned anything from alcohol warning labels?, in *Proceedings of the 1992 Marketing and Public Policy Conference.* P. N. Bloom and R. G. Starr, Jr., eds. Washington, DC, pp. 93–103.

[105]I. Firestone, J. Hankin, J. Ager, J. Sloan, R. Sokol, and S. Martier (1993) What attitudes predict drinking before and during pregnancy? *Alcohol. Clin. Exp. Res.* **17**, 43. (abstract)

[106]J. Hankin, J. Sloan, I. Firestone, J. Ager, R. Sokol, and S. Martier (1993) Birthweight percentile and drinking: a time series analysis. *Alcohol. Clin. Exp. Res.* **17**, 271. (abstract)

[107]J. Hankin, I. Firestone, J. Sloan, J. Ager, R. Sokol, and S. Martier (1993) Listening to the warning again: drinking in the subsequent pregnancy. *Alcohol. Clin. Exp. Res.* **17**, 45. (abstract)

[108]J. Hankin, I. Firestone, J. Sloan, J. Ager, R. Sokol, and S. Martier (1993) The alcohol warning label: impact on knowledge, drinking, and birthweight. *Alcohol. Clin. Exp. Res.* **17**, 270. (abstract)

[109]J. Hankin, J. Sloan, I. Firestone, J. Ager, R. Sokol, S. Martier, and J. Townsend (1993) The alcohol beverage warning label: when did knowledge increase? *Alcohol. Clin. Exp. Res.* **17**, 428–430.

[110]J. Hankin, J. Sloan, I. Firestone, J. Ager, R. Sokol, and S. Martier (1993) A time series analysis of the impact of the alcohol warning label on antenatal drinking. *Alcohol. Clin. Exp. Res.* **17**, 284–289.

[111]J. Hankin, I. Firestone, R. Sokol, S. Martier, J. Ager, and J. Sloan (1992) The "second time around": risk drinking in the subsequent pregnancy. *Alcohol. Clin. Exp. Res.* **16**, 390. (abstract)

[112]J. Hankin, I. Firestone, R. Sokol, J. Ager, and S. Martier (1991) The alcohol beverage warning label: I. Has knowledge changed? *Alcohol. Clin. Exp. Res.* **15**, 385. (abstract)

[113]J. Hankin, I. Firestone, R. Sokol, J. Ager, and S. Martier (1991) The alcohol beverage warning label: II. Determinants of increased knowledge. *Alcohol. Clin. Exp. Res.* **15**, 385. (abstract)

[114]G. Marin (1990) *Awareness of Alcohol and Tobacco Warning Labels Among a Cohort of Hispanics: 1989–1990.* Technical Report No. 3, University of San Francisco Social Psychology Laboratory, pp. 1–36.

[115]G. Marin (1994) Self-reported awareness of the presence of product warning messages and signs by Hispanics in San Francisco. *Public Health Rep.* **109**, 275–283.

[116]D. MacKinnon, M. Pentz, A. Stacy, and K. Taft (1993) *Second Year Effects of the Alcohol Warning Label on Adolescents.* Presentation at American Public Health Association 121st Annual Meeting, October, San Francisco, CA.

[117]T. Prugh (1989) Point-of-purchase health warning notices. *Alcohol Health Res. World* **10**, 36.

[118]A. M. Fenaughty and D. P. MacKinnon (1993) Immediate effects of the Arizona alcohol warning poster. *J. Public Policy Marketing* **12**, 69–77.

[119]R. M. Groves, P. P Beimer, L. E. Lyberg, J. T. Massey, W. L. Nicholls II, and J. Waksberg, eds. (1988) *Telephone Survey Methodology.* Wiley, New York.

[120]J. J. Ray (1983) Reviving the problem of acquiescent response bias. *J. Soc. Psychol.* **121**, 81–96.

[121]T. D. Cook and D. T. Campbell (1978) *Quasi-Experimentation Design and Analysis Issues for Field Settings.* Rand McNally, Chicago.

[122]L. A. Kaskutas (1993) Differential perceptions of alcohol policy effectiveness. *J. Public Health Policy* **14**, 413.

[123]P. Slovic (1987) Perception of risk. *Science* **236**, 280–285.

[124]P. Slovic, B. Fischoff, and S. Lichtenstein (1980) Facts and fears: understanding perceived risk, in *Societal Risk Assessment: How Safe Is Safe Enough?* R. Schwing and W. A. Albers, Jr., eds. Penguin, New York, pp. 181–216.

[125]T. R. Tyler and F. L. Cook (1984) The mass media and judgments of risk: distinguishing impact on personal and societal level judgements. *J. Pers. Soc. Psychol.* **47**, 693–708.

[126]K. H. Beck and A. Frankel (1981) A conceptualization of threat communications and protective health behavior. *Soc. Psychol. Q.* **4**, 204–217.

Cocaine and Injuries

Kenneth Tardiff and Peter Marzuk

Introduction

Compared to the massive literature on the effects of ethanol on injuries, little has been written about cocaine, despite the fact that it is a drug that can produce profound effects on the human mind and body. Most of the literature on cocaine has described the medical complications of cocaine use, such as acute myocardial infarction, cardiac arrhythmias, rupture of the ascending aorta, strokes, seizures, delirium, mood disturbances, psychosis, and other neuropsychiatric complications.[1,2] A brief review of the pharmacology of cocaine should explain how cocaine can impair thinking and performance, which would be expected to increase the risk of injuries, whether accidental or deliberate, as in the case of violence or suicide.

Cocaine hydrochloride appears as a white powder that is usually inhaled nasally or dissolved in water and injected intravenously. The psychoactive effects are gradual when inhaled nasally but the effect is immediate when injected. Cocaine hydrochloride is destroyed if smoked, however the cocaine alkaloid or free base in the form of "crack" is heat-stable and thus can be smoked. The effect of smoking cocaine free base is similar to injecting cocaine since the pulmonary blood supply almost instantaneously carries cocaine to the brain.

Cocaine blocks the presynaptic reuptake of the neurotransmitters norepinephrine and dopamine, thus increasing these neurotransmitters at postsynaptic sites.[1] Increased norepinephrine produces increased heart rate, increased blood pressure, constriction of arteries, and other signs of stimulation of the sympathetic nervous system, which is responsible for a number of medical complications mentioned earlier. Increase of dopamine produces an ini-

From: *Drug and Alcohol Abuse Reviews, Vol. 7: Alcohol, Cocaine, and Accidents*
Ed.: R. R. Watson ©1995 Humana Press Inc., Totowa, NJ

tial euphoria or feeling of extreme well-being. The psychological effect of cocaine is short lived with a subsequent feeling of depression and craving for the drug. The rapid onset of the withdrawal phase results in repetitive use of more cocaine, often until the supply of the drug is exhausted.

Continued administration leads to irritability, suspiciousness, paranoid thinking, and impairment of judgment, even to the extent of psychosis, delirium, and bizarre behavior, including violence.[3] Chronic and/or heavy use of cocaine results in depletion of all neurotransmitters. This may explain the "crash" or feeling of profound depression, lack of energy, and suicidal thoughts following cessation of use of cocaine.[4] The withdrawal phase can last for days. Thus both withdrawal and intoxication from cocaine can produce impairment of judgment, emotions, and behavior.

There is evidence that the ingestion of ethanol with cocaine can produce an active metabolite, cocaethylene, which produces psychological and physical effects similar to cocaine but for a longer duration of time. The half-life of cocaethylene is roughly 2 h, which is twice as long as cocaine. This may be account for toxicity even after cocaine and alcohol levels are negative in blood toxicology reports.[5]

Most studies of emergency room cases or medical examiner cases use measurement of benzoylecgonine, an inactive metabolite of cocaine, as evidence of recent cocaine use. Benzoylecgonine has a half-life of 6–7 h so that a typical dose of cocaine would result in detection of benzoylecgonine for as long as 48 h after the use of cocaine.[6] However, it should be pointed out that detection of benzoylecgonine at autopsy provides evidence only of antemortem use of cocaine and does not allow one to infer dosage, or even duration of use. Although it is widely assumed that heavy, longer term users are at greater risk of fatal injuries, a dose-risk curve has never been established for cocaine. Moreover, cocaine can be conclusively established as a causative risk factor only if those dying in fatal injuries are shown to have high rates of cocaine use compared with suitable population-based controls.

Accidents

The earliest systematic study of cocaine and other drugs detected in motor vehicle accident victims was done by Cimbara and colleagues in Ontario from 1978–1979.[7] Of 484 drivers and pedestrians only one victim (0.2%) was positive for benzoylecgonine, which indicates use of cocaine prior to the accident. He was a 26-yr-old male driver who also had a toxicology positive for ethanol. Overall, the most common drugs found in drivers and pedestrians were cannabinoids (12.2%) and diazepam (3.3%).

As studies were done in the mid-1980s, the percentage of victims reported to have used cocaine before motor vehicle accidents increased. Rogers and colleagues[8] found that the percentage of cocaine-related deaths around Tucson, AZ increased 150% from 1982–1984.[8] Of the 40 cocaine-related deaths in 1984, 25% were motor vehicle accidents and 8% were other accidents. Tardiff and colleagues[9] in New York in 1986 found that only 4% of cocaine-related deaths were motor vehicle accidents and 4% were other types of accidents. The greater number of cocaine-related homicides in New York City probably accounts for motor vehicle accidents representing a smaller percentage of cocaine-related deaths. Williams and colleagues[10] assessed the presence of a number of drugs and alcohol in fatalities involving male drivers ages 15–34 yr in four counties in California in 1983. Recent cocaine use was found in 11% of these drivers, whereas alcohol was found in 70% and marijuana in 37% of cases. Cocaine use was found more frequently among teenage drivers, whereas alcohol was found among drivers 25 yr and older. Marzuk and colleagues[11] examined recent cocaine use among drivers as well as passengers in fatal accidents in New York City from 1984 through 1987. The percentage of benzoylecgonine-positive fatalities among young drivers was 25%, much higher than found by Rogers et al.[8] in California. Roughly half of those positive for recent cocaine use were also positive for ethanol. To test indirectly whether impairment of drivers was associated with recent cocaine use, passengers were used as a comparison group. Of drivers of all ages, 20% were found to be positive for cocaine compared to 14% of passengers. However, this difference did not represent a statistically significant difference.

Wetli and Fishbain[12] focused on cases of cocaine-induced psychosis and sudden death in Miami during a 13-mo period in 1983 and 1984. Of the seven cases, two involved onset of a delirium while driving an automobile and another jumped from a car. One man rammed a van into the front of a house and began running around the neighborhood jumping over fences and pounding on doors before being apprehended by the police and suddenly dying in custody. Another man was snorting cocaine with his girlfriend when he suddenly became violent, claimed that people were after him, and ran to his car. He led the police on a high-speed chase, was apprehended, and suddenly stopped breathing. The passenger who jumped from a car was a young woman who suddenly became violent and paranoid while her boyfriend was driving. Police passing by tried to restrain her and she died shortly afterward by what appeared to be choking or aspiration. The other cases involved violence toward other persons and are described later. One case did involve an accident as a man jumped down a flight of steps while intoxicated with cocaine and died of a ruptured bowel.

It appears that greater numbers of victims in motor vehicle accidents were using cocaine before death in the mid-1980s than earlier in that decade. A few cases of severe cocaine toxicity have been described and found to be directly associated with the fatal accident.[12] Yet there is no definite evidence that impairment by cocaine accounted for driving fatalities in the large medical examiner studies of recent cocaine use.[7-11] We are currently analyzing driver and passenger fatalities, comparing the presence of the active parent compound of cocaine with the presence of only the inactive metabolite benzoylecgonine. This may enable us to look at intoxication at the time of the accident rather than simply having a marker of drug use any time up to 48 h prior to the accident.

Marzuk and colleagues[13] studied 14 Russian roulette deaths by firearms from 1984–1987 in New York. These are not accidents but do represent an extreme form of risk taking. We compared them to firearm deaths that were not certified as homicides. There were no statistically significant differences between the Russian roulette group and the control group in terms of age, gender, or race. The prevalence of recent cocaine use among Russian roulette fatalities (64.3%) was almost twice that of the control group (35.2%). We suspect that cocaine contributes to accidents by impairing judgment and increasing risk taking. It is possible that there is some noncausative link between using cocaine and getting into accidents, such as a certain personality type, but the powerful effects of cocaine on the brain make us doubt that this explains it all.

Violence Toward Others

In the extreme cases of cocaine psychosis and death described by Wetli and Fishbain, there were instances of severe violence toward people.[12] These included a man who was taking cocaine and had a fight with his friend and began to yell, run around, take his clothes off, smash objects, and eventually punch through a glass window and die. Another man used free-base cocaine, then began running down the street with the police chasing him. When he was apprehended, he grabbed hold of an officer's gun and fired it at the police. He was struck on the head a number of times in a struggle and died.

There is evidence that violence among cocaine users is not limited to a few cases of severe violence. In a national telephone hotline in 1993, Roehrich and Gold[14] found that among a group of adolescent cocaine users 27% had been involved in violent behaviors and 13% had been in motor vehicle accidents. Most were polysubstance abusers, predominantly using ethanol, marijuana, and sedative hypnotics. Most of the cocaine users (88%) used the intranasal route.

Studies of patients presenting to emergency rooms also have documented the increased propensity for violence by cocaine users. Brody[15] assessed a subset of 223 patients presenting to an emergency room in Atlanta in a 6-mo period in 1986 and 1987. The subset was identified because the term cocaine was found somewhere in the medical record. There were 37 patients with acute cocaine intoxication and violence. The violence included attacks on persons, destruction of property, or other threatening behaviors that required physical restraint. Other substances of abuse, including alcohol, were commonly used with cocaine. Many of the violent incidents involved extreme exertion, such as running down streets and struggles with the police. Another study of 169 patients tested for drugs in an emergency room in Philadelphia in 1988 showed that cocaine and/or metabolites were present in 91 (53.8%) of patients.[16] Those patients with recent cocaine use were more likely than patients negative for cocaine to have been involved in a violent crime (65.4%), as a perpetrator or victim, or involved in an accident (43.2%), such as a motor vehicle accident or fall. As with other studies cited in this section, other drugs of abuse and alcohol were frequently used with cocaine.

There is some difference of opinion as to how cocaine produces violence. Honer et al.[17] reviewed cases of cocaine abuse presenting to an emergency room in New York for a 7-mo period in 1985 and 1986. They found that patients using crack cocaine were more likely to be psychotic with hallucinations, paranoia, and other delusional thinking, and were more likely than users of other forms of cocaine to injure other persons. They suggested that the more dramatic manifestations with the use of crack cocaine may be owing to the more rapid rise in brain concentration through the pulmonary vasculature. This is questionable since rapid rise in brain concentration would be expected in some of the other methods of administering cocaine such as free-base cocaine smoked or cocaine hydrochloride injected intravenously. These patients did not manifest the same degree of psychosis or violence. Brower et al.[18] studied cocaine users presenting to an emergency room in Michigan. They found that the route of administration (i.e., smoking, intravenous, or intranasal) was not related to the presence of psychosis or violence, but that the amount of cocaine and duration of acute use was related to increased psychosis and violence.

There is evidence that cocaine, particularly prolonged use, may produce violence through its effect on decreasing serotonin.[19] Decreased levels of serotonin have been implicated in violent and suicidal behaviors, particularly those of an impulsive nature.[20–22] Serotonin is an important transmitter probably responsible for inhibition of neuronal activity related to aggressive behavior. Cocaine may deplete the brain of serotonin and produce disinhibition resulting in violence without psychosis or delirium present. Ethanol reduces levels of serotonin.[23] Ethanol is often used with cocaine, so that there may be an additive effect of depletion of serotonin and disinhibited violent behavior with cocaine and ethanol.

Homicide

A number of studies have looked at victims of homicide using medical examiner cases and toxicology for cocaine metabolites to analyze trends in the use of cocaine. It is striking that the percentage of homicide victims with recent cocaine use has gone from very low rates around 1980 to very much increased rates by the end of the decade. Around 1980, studies found that 1–3% of homicide victims had used cocaine the day or two before being murdered.[24-26] By 1986 the percentage of homicide victims positive for cocaine and/or metabolites had risen to almost 20%. Cocaine was second only to ethanol in frequency of detection among homicide victims.[25-27] By 1989 in Atlanta the percentage of homicide victims positive for cocaine metabolites rose to 40%.[28] Tardiff et al.[29] conducted a study of all homicides in New York City in 1990 and 1991. Unlike previous studies, they took into consideration the time interval between injury and death of the victim. A typical dose of cocaine benzoylecgonine leaves the body after 48 h. We excluded from the analysis of benzoylecgonine all cases where the victim lived longer than 48 h so as to avoid false negatives. The overall rate of cases positive for benzoylecgonine and indicating recent cocaine use was 31%.

The problem with using homicide victims to measure recent cocaine use is that the person committing the violent act is not the subject of study. One may speculate that the victims intoxicated with cocaine and/or ethanol may have behaved in a provocative manner or through poor judgment placed themselves in jeopardy. Information about the victims' behavior before being murdered is understandably sketchy. However, Budd[27] found that 20% of victims of violent deaths were found to be acting violently themselves at the time of death and that many of them had been using cocaine and ethanol. Slade et al.[30] assessed 20 medical examiner cases of domestic homicide who were predominantly spouses and lovers in San Francisco from 1985–1988. Toxicology was available for both suspects and victims. They found that 30% of suspects and 15% of victims had evidence of recent cocaine use before the homicide. Ethanol was detected in 70% of suspects and 45% of victims. Although there is an association between cocaine and homicide, the exact relationship of lethal violence and drug use is unknown. For instance, does the use of cocaine and alcohol increase the risk of violence or does domestic violence result in cocaine or alcohol abuse as an attempt to cope with the violence or self-medicate for depression and other psychological distress and suffering?

Some demographic groups have greater proportions of homicide victims with recent use of cocaine than other groups. Earlier studies found that rates of recent cocaine use were increased among Blacks. In New Orleans from 1979–1986, the proportion of cocaine-related homicides increased dramatically, and the population with the greatest increase of cocaine use were young Black males.[25] In the Atlanta area in 1989, Black males and females were more likely than Whites to have recently used cocaine before being murdered, and more likely to die by firearms.[28] In New York in 1990 and 1991, Blacks and Hispanics were almost twice as likely as Whites to have used cocaine before being murdered after controlling for age and gender.[29] Victims ages 25–44 yr were most likely to have cocaine detected at autopsy. Women in this age group were just as likely as men to have had recent cocaine use before death. This is surprising since women in general report less use of cocaine and other drugs than men in society. Women who use cocaine may place themselves in risky situations such as prostitution or in areas where drug dealing and using take place.

Goldstein et al.[31] studied both the setting and the process of buying and selling cocaine and how these may account for the association between cocaine and homicide. They formulated a systemic model of violence caused by cocaine. This involves "the normally aggressive patterns of interaction within the systems of drug use and distribution" (p. 656). Most systemic violence is posited to arise from the exigencies of working or doing business in a black market. Examples of systemic violence include:

1. Territorial disputes between rival dealers;
2. Assaults and homicides committed within particular drug-dealing operations in order to enforce normative codes;
3. Robberies of drug dealers;
4. Elimination of informers;
5. Punishment for selling adulterated or bogus drugs; and
6. Assaults to collect drug-related debts.

Systemic violence may also occur between users, as in cases of disputes over drugs or drug paraphernalia. Goldstein et al.[31] differentiated the systemic events relating cocaine and violence from the pharmacological effects of cocaine-producing violence and impaired judgment described earlier in this chapter. They also excluded from the systemic model violence committed in the process of robbery aimed at obtaining money for cocaine, which they classified as "economic." They looked at 414 homicides in New York in 1988 in which the police at the homicide scene classified these cases using Goldstein et al.'s topology of homicide. There were 218 cases (52.7%) that were drug-related. Of these drug-related cases, 74.3% were classified as systemic and 7.8% were both systemic and psychopharmacological. Of drug-related homicides, 14.2% were classified as owing only to the psychopharmacological effects of cocaine.

One would expect that both the pharmacological and systemic effects apply. There would be a combined effect of the pharmacological effect of cocaine, with irritability and impaired judgment and the dangerous process of buying and selling cocaine. In Memphis, Haruff et al.[26] reported that the police found that cocaine contributed directly to the homicide in 39% of the cases where the drug was detected at autopsy. This involved users being killed by dealers because of bad debts, users being robbed, dealers being killed by users, and vice versa during arguments. They concluded that it was both the dangerous environment as well as the drug-altered behavior of persons under its influence contributing to the homicide.

Suicide

A link between cocaine and suicide has been appreciated for at least 15 yr. In the early 1980s both the number of cocaine-related emergency room visits and deaths increased dramatically.[32] Moreover, 14% of callers to a toll-free cocaine hotline reported having recently attempted suicide.[14] Suicide accounted for 7–15% of all cocaine-related deaths in the early- to mid-1980s.[8,9,27] The San Diego suicide study, one of the most extensive psychological autopsy investigations ever conducted, found that in the early 1980s, 30% of those under the age of 30 yr who committed suicide had a history of cocaine use.[33]

In the mid-1980s a large study of suicide and cocaine in New York found that one in five suicide victims under age 61 had benzoylecgonine detected at autopsy.[9,34] Rates of recent cocaine use were as high as 45% among young male Hispanic victims. Although the study did not use a control group, a contemporaneously conducted household drug survey found a rate of cocaine use in the last 30 d of only 3–5%, which in the context of the medical examiner study suggests that cocaine is a risk factor for suicide.[35]

Preliminary data from the New York City Medical Examiner's Office in 1990 suggest the rate of cocaine use among suicide victims remained as high as it did in 1985, particularly among minority youth.[36] In fact, young age and Black and Hispanic race ethnicity were all independent variables associated with increased detection of cocaine use at autopsy for suicide. Although cocaine use was detected among suicides that had used all types of lethal means, those who used firearms were twice as likely to have used cocaine as those who had used other suicide methods.

The exact mechanism through which cocaine enhances suicide risk is not known. For example, the risk may be greater during the acute intoxication phase several minutes to hours after drug use during which users are apt to be disinhibited, irritable, and paranoid.[37] Others may be more suicidal in the days to weeks after a binge during a withdrawal phase that can involve profound depression.[4] Chronic use of cocaine results in serotonin depletion.[38] A deficiency state involving serotonin has been linked to impulsive suicidal behavior.[39]

A simple pharmacologic explanation for suicide risk is unlikely.[34] It is true that suicide rates among adolescents increased dramatically in the past three decades and many attribute this rise to substance abuse.[40] However, cocaine did not achieve widespread use until the 1980s and suicide rates in the 1980s have not appreciably changed. Thus, this is unlikely that cocaine, *per se,* induces people to commit suicide. More likely, cocaine works with other risk factors to enhance vulnerability to suicide. For instance, many cocaine users are also alcoholics, and alcoholism is known to be strong risk factor for suicide. Cocaine use is often comorbid with other mental disorders, such as depression, anxiety, and schizophrenia, conditions that carry an independent risk for suicide.[41] Some have suggested, for instance, that many cocaine users are self-medicating underlying mental disorders.[42] Chronic substance abusers also experience a wide range of psychosocial stressors that are linked to suicidal behavior, including physical health, marital discord, legal and financial difficulties, and unemployment. Cocaine use is associated with suicide but additional studies are needed to establish both the mechanism of risk and to develop prevention strategies.

Summary and Conclusion

Cocaine is a drug with profound pharmacologic effects on the human mind and body. Its use and the process of buying and selling the drug is entwined in a complex set of social forces that place users and sellers at risk of bodily injury. Cocaine impairs judgment and probably increases risk taking in both the intoxicated and withdrawal state. Studies using medical examiner data show that a substantial proportion of victims of motor vehicle accidents, homicides, and suicides are positive for the metabolites of cocaine. This indicates use of cocaine at least in the day or two prior to the fatal injury. Recent use of cocaine before death is disproportionately increased among the young and the Black and Hispanic populations.

In medical examiner studies, data from emergency departments of hospitals, and data from surveys, there is evidence that cocaine can produce severe violence in cases described in the literature. The number of cases with cocaine-induced violence is convincing but there is no hard evidence that the large number of medical examiner cases of homicide, suicide, or accidents were related to impairment secondary to the pharmacologic effects of cocaine. Could ethanol or other drugs taken with cocaine be responsible for injuries? Could homicides positive for recent cocaine use result from the business of buying and selling cocaine rather than an effect on the behavior of the victim?

Future studies must assess the active form of the drug cocaine and be more sophisticated in terms of methodology. For example, since cocaine is rapidly metabolized within 6 h or so, the interval between injury and death must be considered and cases excluded if the time interval exceeds 6 h so as to avoid false negatives. The intoxicated state should be compared to the withdrawal state in terms of impairment and fatal injuries. Last, demographic and socioeconomic factors must be delineated and studied to determine how they may account for patterns of injury and cocaine use. These sophisticated monitoring projects for cocaine and injury should be conducted and replicated in a variety of geographic areas so as to map the impact of cocaine in the future.

References

[1]L. Cregler and H. Mark (1986) Medical complications of cocaine abuse. *N. Engl. J. Med.* **315,** 1495–1500.

[2]D. Lowenstein, S. Massa, M. Rowbotham, S. Colins, H. McKinney, and R. Simon (1987) Acute neurologic and psychiatric complications associated with cocaine abuse. *Am. J. Med.* **83,** 841–846.

[3]R. Mendoza and B. Miller (1992) Neuropsychiatric disorders associated with cocaine use. *Hosp. Comm. Psychiatry* **43,** 677–680.

[4]F. Gawin and H. Kleber (1986) Abstinence symptomatology and psychiatric diagnosis in cocaine abusers. *Arch. Gen. Psychiatry* **43,** 107–113.

[5]S. Karch (1993) *The Pathology of Drug Abuse.* CRC Press, Boca Raton, FL.

[6]R. Basett (1974) *Disposition of Toxic Drugs and Chemicals in Man,* 2nd ed. Biomedical Publications, Davis, CA.

[7]G. Cimbura, M. Phm, D. Lucas, R. Bennett, R. Warren, and H. Simpson (1982) Incidence and toxicological aspects of drugs detected in 484 fatally injured drivers and pedestrians in Ontario. *J. Forensic Sci.* **27,** 855–867.

[8]J. Rogers, T. Henry, A. Jones, R. Froede, and J. Byers (1986) Cocaine-related deaths in Pima County Arizona, 1982–1984. *J. Forensic Sci.* **31,** 1404–1408.

[9]K. Tardiff, E. Gross, J. Wu, M. Stajic, and R. Millman (1989) Analysis of cocaine-positive fatalities. *J. Forensic Sci.* **34,** 53–63.

[10]A. Williams, M. Peat, D. Crouch, J. Wells, and B. Finkle (1985) Drugs in fatally injured young male drivers. *Public Health Rep.* **100,** 19–25.

[11]P. Marzuk, K. Tardiff, A. Leon, M. Stajic, E. Morgan, and J. Mann (1990) Prevalence of recent cocaine use among motor vehicle fatalities in New York City. *JAMA* **263,** 250–256.

[12]C. Wetli and D. Fishbain (1985) Cocaine-induced psychosis and sudden death in recreational cocaine users. *J. Forensic Sci.* **30,** 873–880.

[13]P. Marzuk, K. Tardiff, D. Smyth, M. Stajic, and A. Leon (1992) Cocaine use, risk-taking, and fatal Russian Roulette. *JAMA* **267,** 2635–2637.

[14]H. Roehrich and M. Gold (1988) 800-COCAINE: origin, significance, and findings. *Yale J. Biol. Med.* **61,** 149–155.

[15]S. Brody (1990) Violence associated with acute cocaine use in patients admitted to a medical emergency department, in *Drugs and Violence: Causes, Correlates and Consequences.* M. De La Rosa, E. Lambert, and B. Gropper, eds. US Department of Health and Human Services, Washington, DC, pp. 44–59.

[16]G. Lindenbaum, S. Carroll, I. Daskal, and R. Kapusnick (1989) Patterns of alcohol and drug abuse in an urban trauma center: the increasing role of cocaine. *J. Trauma* **29,** 1654–1658.

[17]W. Honer, G. Gerwitz, and M. Turey (1987) Psychosis and violence in cocaine smokers. *Lancet* **2,** 451.

[18]K. Brower, F. Blow, and T. Beresford (1988) Forms of cocaine and psychiatric symptoms. *Lancet* **1,** 50.

[19]G. Hanson, L. Matsuda, and J. Gibb (1987) Effects of cocaine on methamphetamine-induced neurochemical changes: characterization of cocaine as a monoamine uptake blocker. *J. Pharmacol. Exp. Ther.* **242,** 507–513.

[20]G. Brown, M. Ebert, P. Goyer, D. C. Jimerson, W. J. Klein, W. E. Bunney, and F. K. Goodwin (1982) Aggression, suicide and serotonin: relationship to CSF amine metabolites. *Am. J. Psychiatry* **136,** 741–746.

[21]L. Lidberg, J. Tuck, M. Asberg, P. Scalia-Tomba, and L. Bertilsson (1985) Homicide, suicide, and CSF 5-HIAA. *Acta Psychiatr. Scand.* **71,** 230–236.

[22]A. Linnolia, M. Virkkunen, M. Scheinin, A. Nuutila, R. Rimon, and F. Goodwin (1983) Low cerebrospinal fluid 5-hydroxyindoleocetic acid concentration differentiates impulsive from nonimpulsive violent behavior. *Life Sci.* **33,** 2609–2614.

[23]J. Collins and W. Schlenger (1988) Acute and chronic effects of alcohol use. *J. Stud. Alcohol* **49,** 516–521.

[24]K. Tardiff, E. Gross, and S. Messner (1986) A study of homicides in Manhattan, 1981. *Am. J. Public Health* **76,** 139–143.

[25]P. Lowry, S. Hassig, R. Gunn, and J. Mathison (1988) Homicide victims in New Orleans: recent trends. *Am. J. Epidemiol.* **128,** 1130–1136.

[26]R. Harruff, J. Francisco, S. Elkins, A. Phillips, and G. Fernandez (1988) Cocaine and homicide in Memphis and Shelby County: an epidemic of violence. *J. Forensic Sci.* **33,** 1231–1237.

[27]R. Budd (1989) Cocaine abuse and violent death. *Am. J. Drug Alcohol Abuse* **15,** 375–382.

[28]R. Hanzlick and G. Gowitt (1991) Cocaine metabolite detection in homicide victims. *JAMA* **265,** 760,761.

[29]K. Tardiff, P. Marzuk, A. Leon, C. Hirsch, M. Stajic, L. Portera, and N. Hartwell (1994) *Homicide in New York City: cocaine use and firearms. JAMA* **272,** 43–46.

[30]M. Slade, L. Daniel, and C. Heisler (1991) Application of forensic toxicology to the problem of domestic violence. *J. Forensic Sci.* **36,** 708–713.

[31]P. Goldstein, H. Brownstein, P. Ryan, and P. Bellucci (1989) Crack and homicide in New York City, 1988: a conceptually based event analysis. *Contemp. Drug Probl.* **16,** 651–687.

[32]National Institute on Drug Abuse (1987) *Trends in Drug Abuse Related Hospital Emergency Room Episodes and Medical Examiner Cases for Selected Drugs.* US Department of Health and Human Services, Washington, DC.

[33]R. Fowler, C. Rich, and D. Young (1986) San Diego suicide study, II: substance abuse in young cases. *Arch. Gen. Psychiatry* **43,** 962–965.

[34]P. Marzuk and J. Mamm (1988) Suicide and substance abuse. *Psychiatr. Ann.* **18,** 639–645.

[35]New York State Division of Substance Abuse Services (1988) *Statewide Household Survey of Substance Abuse, 1986: Illicit Substance Use Among Hispanic Adults in New York State.* Author, Albany, NY.

[36]P. Marzuk, K. Tardiff, A. Leon, C. Hirsch, M. Stajic, L. Portera, and N. Hartwell. *Racial-Ethnic Differences in Urban Suicide: The Role of Guns and Cocaine,* manuscript submitted.

[37]F. Gawin and E. Ellinwood (1988) Cocaine and other stimulants: actions, abuse and treatment. *N. Engl. J. Med.* **318,** 1173–1182.

[38]C. Dackis and M. Gold (1985) New concepts in cocaine addiction: the dopamine depletion hypothesis. *Neurosci. Biobehav. Rev.* **9,** 469–477.

[39]G. Brown and F. Goodwin (1986) Cerebrospinal fluid correlates of suicide attempts and aggression. *Ann. NY Acad. Sci.* **487,** 175–188.

[40]F. Crumley (1990) Substance abuse and adolescent suicidal behavior. *JAMA* **263,** 3051–3056.

[41]A. Roy (1983) Risk factors for suicide in psychiatric patients. *Arch. Gen. Psychiatry* **40,** 971–974.

[42]E. Khantzian (1985) The self medication hypothesis of additive disorders: focus on heroin and cocaine dependence. *Am. J. Psychiatry* **142,** 1259–1264.

Community Approaches to Prevention of Alcohol- Related Accidents

Harold D. Holder, Joel W. Grube, Paul J. Gruenewald, Robert F. Saltz, Andrew J. Treno, and Robert B. Voas

Tradition of Community-Level Prevention Programs

Health professionals concerned with the prevention of chronic diseases have accumulated over 20 yr of experience in programs designed to reduce cardiovascular disease (CVD). Some of these studies were carried out in clinical settings or in worksites.[1,2] Other studies in CVD prevention were directed at the entire populations in communities and involved comprehensive approaches combining community organization and multichannel health education.[3-7] These earlier studies represent a rich source of both technical expertise and practical experience that alcohol problem prevention professionals should consider before they design similar projects. However, because most knowledge of community-based public health interventions derives from programs to reduce high-risk medical conditions, the relevance of the medical trials for the management, design, and implementation of alcohol problem prevention should not be automatically assumed.[8,9] For these reasons, the development of a comprehensive community-based program for prevention of alcohol-related injuries and deaths

From: *Drug and Alcohol Abuse Reviews, Vol. 7: Alcohol, Cocaine, and Accidents*
Ed.: R. R. Watson ©1995 Humana Press Inc., Totowa, NJ

requires special attention to linkage of public education and community organizers with agencies involved in regulatory and environmental policies. Strategies used in such interventions will require many innovations beyond those used for other health domains to insure their relevance to alcohol-related trauma.

Community-based alcohol prevention efforts are very rare. A majority of prevention programs have been targeted at children and adolescents and have been specifically concerned with knowledge about alcohol, attitudes and values about drinking, and self-reported drinking (particularly drinking initiation). Some of these projects have had success in increasing knowledge levels and changing attitudes and values, and a few have reduced the level of self-reported drinking and/or drinking initiation.[10] Pentz et al.[11] reported lower rates of drinking initiation following a comprehensive school-based training, but we do not know the relationship between drinking initiation and the risk of alcohol-related auto crashes and other alcohol trauma for adolescent drinkers.

Such school-based-only approaches contrast with true comprehensive community prevention programs in four ways. First, school-based projects have focused on drinking initiation and drinking in general and not alcohol-related trauma. Second, most such programs emphasize the role of education and training to modify individual student choice behavior rather than changes in the structural features of the community about alcohol. Third, these projects typically target only part of the total community population, i.e., children and adolescents. Although these adolescents will become adults and move into the larger community, by far the greatest number of alcohol-related trauma involves adults who are not included in the school-based population. Finally, other research suggests the limited ability of school-based educational approaches by themselves to reduce community-level alcohol-related problems. Such programs need the complementary support of other strategies.[12,13]

Even with the few community prevention projects that have addressed the total community population (including children, adolescents, and adults) and/or have addressed community level problems, none of them can be characterized by all of the following:

1.   The development of a careful baseline planning and preintervention period with well-defined community-level alcohol problems as targets;
2.   A long-term implementation and monitoring period;
3.   A followup or summative evaluation of changes in target problems; and
4.   A scientifically determined successful result or change in the target(s) that can be confidently attributed to the intervention.

Thus, one must conclude that there has been no community-based alcohol prevention project to date that has produced long-term reductions in community-level alcohol problems.[10,14]

Examples of Previous Community-Wide Alcohol Problem Prevention Strategies

Most previous community prevention efforts for alcohol problems can be characterized by one of the following case studies. However, few efforts to reduce community-level alcohol problems have been undertaken over the past 30 yr that meet even minimum conditions for scientific evaluation, i.e., can be considered an example of a community prevention controlled trial.

One early community experiment was undertaken in Finland from 1951–1953 to alter the availability of alcohol in rural areas (*see* Kuusi[15] for full discussion of the experiment and results). No legal sale of alcohol had taken place in rural areas in Finland since 1902. The law required that all alcohol sales be made by the State Alcohol Monopoly (ALKO) and then only in cities. Thus, rural residents had to visit cities for their alcohol. The market towns, Ikaalinen, Nokia, and Jarvenpaa, in south western and central Finland were selected as the experimental towns where a state-controlled beer and wine retail bottle store would be established. Comparison towns were Ruovesi and Myllykoski. The project evaluation found that:

1. Frequency of drinking among men, but not the overall number of people actually drinking, increased in the test communities;
2. The percentage of drinkers among youth and women did not increase;
3. Both wine and beer increased in use as the beverage of choice with a corresponding reduction in spirits;
4. Illicit alcohol use was reduced;
5. Little change was observed in the quantities consumed per occasion and, thus, there was no reduction in frequency of drunkenness;
6. There were declines in the number of visits to cities in all experimental towns; and
7. Even with the increased availability of beer and wine, such beverages remained a small part of alcohol consumed leading to intoxication.

One of the earliest prevention efforts for community-level prevention of alcohol problems in the United States occurred in California in the mid-1970s. This program, modeled after the three-city Stanford Heart Disease Project,[4] also called for a three-community prevention effort in which one community received community action and focus group communication/ reinforcement and mass media; a second community received the mass media only; and a third control community received no special program. Budget cuts in the evaluation and political interventions limited the mass media messages to those deemed acceptable by the state of California who sponsored the program (i.e., those counter to the interests of the alcoholic beverage industry were excluded) and changed the basic protocol of the project midstream. In the end, the evaluation was reduced to three waves of household surveys concerning recognition of the mass media and other education programs, attitudes and values about drinking, and self-reports of personal drinking patterns. The conclusions of evaluators were that there were some signs of increased awareness and knowledge about alcohol issues, that respondents in the target communities could recognize the campaign's commercials (a majority could interpret the desired preventative message), but that there was no evidence of reductions in drinking behavior and particularly heavy, high-risk drinking.[8,16]

Rootman and Moser[17] and Ritson[18] described a World Health Organization project begun in 1977 to study ways of improving community response to alcohol problems among communities in Mexico, Zambia, and Scotland. The study utilized a series of community epidemiological and social service/health agency surveys. In each study site, community organizing activities were undertaken at the local level and supported by national policy-setting activities. The local emphasis in each country differed. In the Edinburgh metropolitan area, the project contributed to the planning of an ongoing Council of Community Agencies to improve community response to alcohol problems. Some changes in service availability were documented. In a district of Mexico City, the project's activities contributed to efforts to recruit male professionals and women's organizations to discuss alcohol problems. The efforts for males failed. The women's efforts resulted in the formation of mutual support groups of wives of heavy drinkers. The Zambian project attempted to establish community action groups in three study communities but these groups ceased to function when project personnel left.

Another American community-based prevention project was undertaken in San Francisco in 1983.[19] Researchers worked with substance abuse services to convene a series of half-day community workshops attended by representatives of local agencies and interest groups including: the city council, the mayor's office, the public schools, the public defender's office, alcohol and mental health treatment organizations, local newspapers, unions, the State Department of Alcoholic Beverage Control, and youth organizations. The workshops had two purposes: to increase local leaders' awareness of the extent of alcohol-related problems and to give them an environmental view of such problems; and to develop working groups to attack specific problems with detailed action.[19-21] As part of the campaign, the Community Substance Abuse Services compiled a *San Francisco Fact Book* detailing the history of, policies toward, and responsibilities for alcohol abuse in the city and county of San Francisco. A second product was the direct involvement of workshop participants in developing written community prevention initiatives.[22] One working group sought to prevent a change in local ordinances that would allow the sale of alcohol to motorists stopping in gasoline stations. The work of the group stimulated members of the San Francisco Board of Supervisors to become interested in implementing a training program for bartenders and to establish server-training as an essential part of the hospitality business in the city. Other task forces were created, including one to work against the sale of alcohol to minors and one to undertake a media project to disseminate prevention information. The San Francisco project documented the potential interest of community leaders in alcohol problems and the community action groups to stimulate change. There was no evaluation of changes in alcohol problems associated with this community effort and, thus, such final outcomes are unknown.

In 1981, Giesbrecht began a test of community prevention efforts to reduce high-risk drinking levels. Three towns in the province of Ontario, Canada were used, one test and two control communities.[23] In the test community, the project goal was to reduce the drinking of these drinkers to under 12 drinks a week. A first step in the program was to establish an awareness among community members of their drinking level as individuals and of the town as a whole using posters and pamphlets. Their awareness enabled them to compare the current drinking level of the community with an ideal "safe drinking" level, both for individuals and for the town in the aggregate. A special target of this educational effort was problem drinkers, defined as those who consume at least 28 drinks a week, who have done so for some time, and who are not aware that this level of consumption puts them at risk. Researchers found that 80% of the people who drink at or below this level reported no significant alcohol problems. The results of the program, utilizing community pre- and postproject surveys and time series analysis of alcohol sales in all three communities, showed no significant change in reported consumption among the heavy drinking group or in community-level alcohol consumption.[24]

A 2½-yr community prevention demonstration project was undertaken in New Zealand between October 1982 and March 1985, sponsored by the Alcoholic Liquor Advisory Council (ALAC) and the Medical Research Council of New Zealand. The program included a paid mass media campaign and use of community organization. Four experimental communities were utilized. All four were exposed to the mass media campaign and two of the four also participated in the community organization. Two reference communities were used as controls. The major focus of this experiment was on social policy concerning regulation of alcoholic beverages. The objectives were to increase support for relevant public health policies concerning alcohol as well as personal moderation in the use of alcohol. The program was designed to increase appropriate alcohol policies by organizations such as city councils and hospital boards. Increased voluntary use of bar-staff server training by licensed establishments and increased involvement of police in the program were implemented. The policy areas that received the most public attention were alcohol availability and advertising. Price received less attention because it was seen as being out of the control of the community. In each of the intensive intervention communities, a local person was recruited as a community organizer on a full-time basis using funds from ALAC. Project evaluation, based on before-and-after surveys, found that public support for control policies on advertising, availability of alcohol, and prices held steady in the treatment communities but dropped in the reference communities amidst a national trend toward greater support for liberalization and reduction of government control.[9,25,26]

Under a cooperative agreement between the Centers for Disease Control (CDC) and the National Institute on Alcohol Abuse and Alcoholism (NIAAA), the Rhode Island Department of Health began a 5-yr community prevention trial in Rhode Island in 1984. The project had the objective of reducing alcohol-related trauma and violence. The treatment community (Woonsocket) was randomly selected from three candidate Rhode Island towns. Prevention efforts in the treatment community were targeted at retail beverage establishments, police, and general community. Interventions at retail establishments were to train servers and licensed establishment owners/managers to adopt responsible sales and service policies and to reduce the number of intoxicated patrons. Police interventions were to increase enforcement of driving under the influence (DUI) laws as well as selective enforcement of server liability using plainclothes detectives. Community level activities included increased publicity about drinking and driving, a program to offer rides for drinking drivers, and employee assistance efforts to foster employer policies against drinking on the job and to reduce alcohol-impaired job performance.

By the end of the demonstration project, after 18 mo of baseline study and 30 mo of intervention, the following objectives were achieved:

1. Written policies for responsible alcohol service were adopted by 100% of off-premise establishments and 79% of on-premise establishments.

2. The program trained 388 sales and service personnel in the techniques for responsible alcohol service representing nearly 61% of servers employed in the community.
3. All members of the Woonsocket police force had received training in recognizing and measuring intoxication, the role of alcohol in police work, police liability in dealing with intoxicated citizens, and on-scene investigation of motor vehicle crashes.
4. The police department had initiated 73 sobriety checkpoints, 47 additional radar patrols, and 11 selective enforcement patrols covering 300 visits to liquor establishments.

Several process indicators suggest that the gatekeepers responded favorably to the interventions. A posttest of servers done 12–18 mo after the training showed changes in attitudes and behavior. The police carried out a vigorous enforcement campaign; arrest data show that alcohol-related arrests increased in Woonsocket, whereas the other two communities showed level or decreasing rates.

Types of Prevention Programs

Most community-based alcohol problem prevention strategies fall into one or more of the following types.

The Individual's Alcohol Use

Historically, the most frequent approach to alcohol problem prevention has focused on individual-level risk factors.

School-Based Alcohol Education

This orientation usually emphasizes prevention of youthful drinking and interventions to prevent problems later in life. Many of these programs are school-based alcohol education programs, and have focused on giving the facts about alcohol use, decision-making skills, peer resistance training, and parents' education.[10,11,27–29]

The Mass Media

In the 1970s there were several efforts to educate the general public about the importance of moderate drinking. A 3-yr demonstration project in California that promoted responsible drinking through the mass media and community organizations showed some increase in awareness but no change in attitudes or behavior.[8] A review of 15 mass media campaigns reveals that some campaigns were effective in changing some audience attributes (knowledge, attitudes, or behavior) some of the time.[30] However, it can be argued for both alcohol and drug media education[31] that no adequate test has occurred of the potential for public education, especially in the context of a comprehensive program that integrates environmental and regulatory changes with educational approaches.

Environmental Approaches to Community Prevention

Most community-level alcohol prevention programs have focused on educational and/or mass media approaches. In contrast, an environmental approach seeks to change the social mechanisms that influence the availability of alcoholic beverages, including not only physical availability (e.g., the regulation of types of beverages sold, minimum age, density of alcohol outlets), but also economic availability or price of alcohol relative to income and other goods,[32] and social availability, including the normative climate regarding alcohol consumption.

There is evidence to show that changes in environmental (usually regulatory) factors can reduce the level of consumption and alcohol-related problems. For example, Gruenewald and colleagues[33,34] found positive associations among regulatory activities of states, retail availability, and alcohol sales. Rush et al.[35] found a positive association among retail availability of alcohol, alcohol consumption, and alcohol-related morbidity and mortality. These analyses suggest that government policies that restrict the availability of alcohol will reduce per capita consumption and, indirectly, lower alcohol-related damage. In addition, Holder and Blose[36] used an interrupted time series analysis in a quasi-experimental design on alcohol-related crash data in North Carolina following the legalization of liquor-by-the-drink (LBD). They found statistically significant increases in crash rates in counties that permitted LBD and no changes in matched comparison counties that did not legalize LBD.[37] Responsible beverage service programs that focus on providing training and on implementing policies to reduce service to intoxicated patrons also appear to be effective in reducing heavy drinking.[38,39] These studies along with many others[40] as well as cross-cultural analyses from other countries[41] are evidence that environmental factors affect both consumption levels (which are shown to be related to alcohol-related problems) and alcohol abuse. After reviewing studies from the United States and other countries, Room[42] concluded that alcohol controls can affect the rates of alcohol-related problems.

Environmental Influences on the Individual's Behavior

The most general environmental influences are *formal and informal* prescriptions and proscriptions regarding drinking. Those areas most relevant to alcohol problem prevention include laws pertaining to alcohol-impaired driving and to the service of alcohol and the less formal normative environment created by the mass media. Some examples follow.

Alcohol-Impaired Driving

Public attention devoted to the driving while intoxicated (DWI) problem during the last decade has probably helped to reduce alcohol-related fatal crashes.[43] Some enforcement programs[44-46] have produced reductions in crashes. However, increased enforcement of DWI laws and increases in penalties for driving under the influence have not consistently reduced overall community-level drinking and driving or alcohol-related crashes. For example, in Maine and Massachusetts, increased penalties for DWI did not correlate with decreases in arrests or crashes for the 3 yr following the change in legislation. It may be that the public perception of enforcement of these laws and swift punishment are central to a decrease in DWI.[47,48]

Dram Shop or Server Liability

Server liability refers to the legal responsibility of someone who serves alcohol (usually in a retail establishment), including civil responsibility for damage and injury caused by a patron served while intoxicated who later causes damage or injury as well as criminal liability for service to an underage person. Since Prohibition, most server liability laws (often called dramshop laws) have been used as the basis for individual litigation to obtain damages, not as public prevention policy. However, Mosher[49] suggested that server liability can have a preventive function.

Responsible Beverage Service

The most recent research that has manipulated drinking contexts or serving practices arises from the interest in server intervention. Here the goal is to reduce a customer's likelihood of intoxication or DWI through a combination of revised management and serving practices, server training, and changes in the physical environment. One of the first evaluations of server intervention,[38,50,51] using a Navy enlisted club that implemented a comprehensive server intervention program, found a reduction in customer blood alcohol concentration (BAC) with no change in a comparison club. In a similar study, Russ and Geller[52] employed research assistants who posed as intoxicated patrons at two bars where approximately half of the staff had been trained. By recording the frequency and type of interventions used by the servers, they were able to show that the trained servers intervened in some way significantly more than did untrained servers. An attempted application of server intervention techniques to noncommercial contexts also has been described.[53]

Community Systems Model
for Alcohol-Related Accident Prevention

A number of community factors give rise to alcohol-induced trauma. Holder[54] identified a number of variables that interact to produce alcohol-related injuries and deaths. Alcohol availability, drinks per occasion, risk behavior such as driving, norms about drinking, and so on, interact to produce such problems. Holder[55] described causal relationships between alcohol use and trauma and environmental factors in a community system. This model identified the most significant factors and domains in a community that should be addressed by prevention interventions or recognized as contributing to problem events.

Example of a Comprehensive
Community Prevention Trial
to Reduce Alcohol-Related Injuries

The Prevention Research Center, Berkeley, CA, is conducting a 5-yr prevention trial sponsored by the NIAAA. This is an example of a long-term research-based, community-based prevention effort and is now in the initial stages of implementation. The purpose of this prevention trial is to implement and evaluate comprehensive interventions to reduce: alcohol-related traffic crashes including injuries and fatalities; and alcohol-related nontraffic fatalities and unintentional injuries including burns, drownings, and falls.

Five interacting and supportive prevention components are being implemented. Each addresses part of a conceptual model of alcohol-related trauma and each has its own specialized data collection procedures that allow a component-specific evaluation of implementation and proximal outcomes. The components are:

1. A Community Knowledge, Values, and Mobilization Component, which consists of working with existing community coalitions in the experimental communities to implement specific interventions and developing an integrated public awareness and education program that supports overall goals and those of individual components, including concern about alcohol-related trauma, the relationship of BAC and impairment as related to increased risk of death or injury, and skills in estimating BAC.

2. A Responsible Beverage Service Component, which includes training of servers and owner/managers of on-premise alcohol outlets to identify intoxicated and/or underage customers in bars and restaurants and to develop and implement beverage service policies that reduce the probability of customers becoming intoxicated or of DWI.

3. An Underage Drinking Component, which is concerned with issues of access and sales of alcohol to minors. This component involves several interventions, including:
   a. Mass media education about issues of youth drinking and access to alcohol;
   b. Parent training and networking to reduce access to alcohol in the home and improve parental supervision of adolescent activities;
   c. Development and implementation of store policies and training of off-premise alcohol clerks to reduce sales to minors; and
   d. Increased enforcement of underage possession and sales laws.
4. A Risk of Drinking and Driving Component, which increases the actual and perceived risk of apprehension rate of drivers who are under the influence of alcohol. This component consists of increasing DWI efficiency through training enforcement officers in new techniques for identifying DWI drivers and the use of passive alcohol sensors to increase the probability of detection.
5. An Access to Alcohol Component, which includes the use of local zoning powers and other municipal control of outlet density to reduce the availability of alcohol that contributes to alcohol problems.

The research design is quasi-experimental with three pairs of treatment and comparison communities: one pair in northern California, one in southern California, and one in South Carolina. The first year was a baseline data collection and planning phase involving a combination of community and emergency room surveys as well as the use of archival records. Years 2 through 4 are intervention phases that make use of a process evaluation and media-based feedback to the community to enhance program effects. The final project year focuses on:

1. Outcome evaluation including the analysis of community-level crash and accident data;
2. Process evaluation of the total project and component implementation; and
3. The institutionalization of the community program components in order to ensure continuity after the research is completed.

The specific outcome measures for this project are alcohol-related traffic crashes and nontraffic trauma.

Alcohol-Related Traffic Crashes

Alcohol is implicated in up to 50% of fatal crashes in the United States. Almost 80% of fatal crashes occur between 8 PM and 4 AM. Each year nearly 560,000 people are injured in alcohol-related crashes and about 43,000 sustain serious injuries.[56–58] In addition, crashes are the leading cause of death for young people under 25. Those under 25 are involved in alcohol-related crashes at higher percentages than expected given their proportion in the driving population.[56,58,59] Nearly 70% of young adults (ages 20–24) who died in traffic crashes were in alcohol-related crashes. Thus, alcohol-related crashes are a significant public health problem, are a natural target for a community prevention study, and have been extensively studied in past research.

A large research literature exists discussing the measurement issues for alcohol-related traffic crashes. Ideally, the BAC of every driver in each crash would be determined. Such measures would provide baseline data for both risk of crash by various BAC levels by age and gender and also provide a consistent standard for monitoring temporal changes in alcohol involvement. However, both cost issues and legal issues of protecting individual rights and legal liability prevent these measures from being routinely collected by law enforcement officers. In most states, crash report forms are used by officers to record judgments whether alcohol was involved in the crash (e.g., driver was drinking), but this coding has obvious measurement problems that prevent it from being utilized as a primary dependent measure. However, officer reports are often consistent with other surrogates for alcohol involvement and are used by some researchers as a dependent measure[60] or as supplements to other measures.[61] Fatal crashes are related to a high percentage of alcohol-related driving and are preferred by some as a surrogate.[62] However, fatal crashes are infrequent enough in many states, and certainly in most communities, to provide insufficient observations and are often unstable over time. Thus, the measure preferred by most traffic researchers is single-vehicle nighttime crashes (i.e., those with only one moving vehicle and occurring between 8 PM and 4 AM). This measure provides more observations per time unit than fatal crashes, has been shown to include a significant number of alcohol-involved drivers,[63–65] and has been shown to be sensitive to changes in alcohol use and availability in studies of minimum purchase age,[66,67] changes in spirits availability,[61] and changes in beverage server liability.[68]

Nontraffic Trauma

Alcohol-related nontraffic unintentional trauma also has a substantial prevalence. Falls, drownings, and burns are the second, third, and fourth leading causes of unintentional death in the United States. With an aggregate incidence rate of 11 deaths per 100,000 annually, these causes of death trail behind rates observed for the leading cause of unintentional death, traffic-related fatalities (18.2/100,000).[69] Deaths owing to falls occur at an annual rate of 5.5/100,000 individuals. Injuries are estimated to occur at the much higher rate of 6700/100,000.[70,71] Of the three sources of unintentional injury and death discussed in this section, alcohol involvement in the case of falls is best documented. (*See* Holder[54] for a theoretical discussion of alcohol's involvement in nontraffic-related trauma.) Deaths owing to drownings occur at an annual rate of 3/100,000.[72] Studies of this cause of death have focused on four water sport activities, swimming/surfing,[73,74] boating,[74,75] fishing,[73,76] and scuba/skin diving.[77] Emergency room studies[78] suggest that alcohol involvement in burn injuries can be found in about 18% of cases. The high rate of reported injuries (as opposed to fatalities) for falls and burns (7123/100,000) suggests that these outcomes may be profitably measured at the community level.

Although knowledge of the contribution of alcohol to nontraffic trauma is not as complete or systematic as that of traffic trauma, these estimates provide evidence of significant involvement that supports the importance of such trauma as a target in a prevention trial. The measurement of nontraffic alcohol-related trauma involves a consideration of both fatal and nonfatal injuries. For nontraffic fatalities, the BAC distribution of all deaths caused by unintentional nontraffic injury will be obtained at least annually from the local county coroner in each experimental and comparison site. However, nonfatal unintentional trauma presents a special problem. Rarely do hospital emergency rooms or even trauma centers collect BAC levels on every patient and even so, triage decision making (sending the most seriously injured to such centers) introduces a selection bias into such systematic measures. Thus, such information is usually collected only when there is a medical indication that alcohol may be involved and to assist the treatment protocol, not as a means to establish alcohol-related rates. Therefore, time sampling as a procedure to collect trauma events experienced in the communities along with self-reports to triangulate on the prevalence of alcohol-related trauma experienced are necessary.

This project involves five phases. Phase 1 of any community prevention program should be dedicated to baseline data collection and detailed project planning. The remaining phases are operational periods and are devoted to carrying out action programs. Phase 2 is to complete community mobilization and to the initial implementation of interventions. Phases 3 and 4 involve comprehensive intervention implementation. The final phase, Phase 5, should be concerned with project evaluation and the institutionalization of programs in the community. A more detailed description of the project phases is provided.

Phase 1

No prevention program interventions are initiated during the baseline period. Rather, this phase is for collection of baseline data (before any intervention) on alcohol-related trauma and other outcomes. Before any interventions or prevention activities are begun, the specific details of prevention interventions in the treatment community must be planned by the participating community coalitions and organizations with technical assistance of the research team. This long-term planning includes the development of procedures for incorporating community participation and pretesting of the initial program delivery and data collection procedures. No extensive mobilization of the community occurs during this period, as this is the time for discussions and planning with the local coalition and key community informants. Some news coverage may occur if meetings are not closed, but no purposeful interventions by the project should be undertaken. The data collection provides baseline as well as formative research for developing local awareness and support.

Phase 2

This year is an initial implementation phase. The first 6 mo should be concerned with community mobilization and education and preintervention baseline for specific interventions (e.g., server training and retail clerk training). Public information may be the first activity to be undertaken by the project to promote community organization and participation in the project, to increase the awareness and concern of the general public about alcohol, and to develop public support for the environmental strategies to be utilized. Initial intervention activities also are implemented in Phase 2. Preintervention data are collected during the first 6 mo just prior to the implementation of the planned interventions during this phase.

Phase 3

During the comprehensive implementation phase, there are additional intervention specific training, other implementation activities, and continued monitoring of the community. All interventions are underway and functioning. Data collection should be of two types: continued monitoring of alcohol-related trauma and administration of community surveys; and collection of post-initial implementation component process/outcome information. Project and component-specific information is collected to document progress/activity (i.e., provide a historical record of the project) as well as provide feedback to the project staff in making necessary improvements and modifications. This phase is concerned with building additional public support and awareness of the program and its goals.

Phase 4

The reinforcement of comprehensive intervention continues activities from Phase 3 and includes "booster activities" to maintain or rekindle interest in the interventions and community coalitions organized to implement them. Data collection, both process and outcome, are continued. Institutionalization efforts are begun and intensified if necessary.

Phase 5

The institutionalization and outcome/intervention assessment phase includes community incorporation of desired program elements, continued community monitoring, and final overall evaluation of the project. Program incorporation by the community is the process in which prevention activities (desired by the community) are established within existing local structures to be continued after outside funding and technical support are ended. Monitoring of alcohol-related trauma and community surveys may be continued through the first half of this phase. Prevention component process and outcome documentation is also continued. Overall program effectiveness evaluation is completed using the primary outcome measures. In addition, intervention component documentation and evaluation and the project history are completed.

Conclusion

A number of phases and steps have been identified for undertaking community-based prevention trials.[79-81] Such discussions share common concepts and approaches. Each highlights key steps and decision points. These discussions all share some of the following, which are directly relevant to the prevention of alcohol-related injuries and deaths:

1. Prevention trials are research projects and as such are driven by (based on) prior research. That is, they utilize in a formal and systematic fashion basic research concerning risk factors and potential intervention points to reduce a specific problem.
2. As research projects, community prevention trials to reduce alcohol-related injuries and deaths are to be subjected to the same scientific rigor as would be expected of basic research projects.
3. Community prevention trials are a natural progression from basic research to application, generally aimed at reducing the incidence and prevalence of health problems.
4. Although based on basic research, prevention trials are concerned with the public health and welfare, and their purpose is to develop the means to reduce problems.

Community prevention trials can become the "living laboratory" tests of the prevention research findings from basic risk studies as well as pilot or small-scale research and scientific prevention program evaluation. Such trials also provide opportunities for communities to put into practice the

findings from alcohol prevention research, particularly to reduce accidental alcohol-related trauma.

Acknowledgment

Research and preparation of this article were supported, in part, by the
National Institute on Alcohol Abuse and Alcoholism Research Center grant
AA06282 to the Prevention Research Center, Pacific Institute for Research
and Evaluation and AA 09146 (jointly funded by the Center for Substance
Abuse and the National Institute on Alcohol Abuse and Alcoholism).

References

[1]M. Kornitzer, D. Dramaix, F. Kittel, and G. Debaker (1980) The Belgian heart
disease prevention project: changes in smoking habits after two years of intervention.
Prev. Med. **9,** 496–503.

[2]R. Benfari (1981) The multiple risk factor intervention trial, III: the model for
intervention. *Prev. Med.* **10,** 426–442.

[3]R. Carlaw, M. Mittlemark, N. Bracht, and R. Luepker (1984) Organization for a
community cardiovascular health program: experiences from the Minnesota Heart Health
Program. *Health Educ. Q.* **11(3),** 243–252.

[4]J. Farquhar, P. D. Wood, H. Breitrose, W. L. Haskell, A. J. Meyer, N. Maccoby, J.
K. Alexander, B. W. Brown, A. L. McAlister, J. D. Nash, and M. P. Stern (1977) Community education for cardiovascular health. *Lancet* **1,** 1192–1195.

[5]T. Lasater, D. Abrams, L. Artz, P. Beaudin, L. Cabrera, J. Elder, et al. (1984) Lay
volunteer delivery of a community-based cardiovascular risk factor change experiment:
the Pawtucket experiment, in *Behavioral Health: A Handbook of Health Enhancement
and Disease Prevention.* J. Matarazzo, N. Miller, S. Weiss, J. Herd, and S. Weiss, eds.
Wiley, New York, pp. 1166–1170.

[6]D. Murray (1986) Dissemination of community health promotion programs: the
Fargo-Moorhead heart health program. *J. School Health* **56(9),** 375–381.

[7]P. Puska, A. Nissinen, J. Tuomilehto, J. Salonen, K. Koskela, A. McAlister, T.
Kottke, N. Maccoby, and J. Farquhar (1985) The community-based strategy to
prevent coronary heart disease: conclusions from the ten years of the North Karelia
project. *Annu. Rev. Public Health* **6,** 147–193.

[8]L. M. Wallack and D. C. Barrows (1982–1983) Evaluating primary prevention: the
California "Winners" alcohol program. *Int. Q. Commun. Health Educ.* **3(4),** 307–336.

[9]S. Casswell and L. Gilmore (1989) An evaluated community action project on alcohol. *J. Stud. Alcohol* **50(4),** 339–346.

[10]J. Moskowitz (1989) The primary prevention of alcohol problems: a critical review
of the research literature. *J. Stud. Alcohol* **50(1),** 54–88.

[11]M. A. Pentz, J. H. Dwyer, D. P. MacKinnon, B. R. Flay, W. B. Hansen, E. Y.
Wang, and C. Anderson-Johnson (1989) A multicommunity trial for primary prevention of adolescent drug abuse. *JAMA* **261(22),** 3259–3266.

[12]A. L. Mauss, R. H. Hopkins, R. A. Weisheit, and K. A. Kearney (1988) The problematic prospects for prevention in the classroom: should alcohol education programs
be expected to reduce drinking by youth? *J. Stud. Alcohol* **49,** 51–61.

[13]M. Klitzner, M. Vegega, and P. J. Gruenewald (1988) An empirical examination of the assumptions underlying youth drinking/driving prevention programs. *Eval. Program Plann.* **11(3)**, 219–235.

[14]H. D. Holder (1992) What is a community and what are implications for prevention trials for reducing alcohol problems, in *Community Prevention Trials for Alcohol Problems: Methodological Issues.* H. D. Holder and J. M. Howard, eds. Praeger, Westport, CT, pp. 15–33.

[15]P. Kuusi (1957) *Alcohol Sales Experiment in Rural Finland.* The Finnish Foundation for Alcohol Studies, Helsinki.

[16]L. M. Wallack and D. C. Barrows (1981) *Preventing Alcohol Problems in California: Evaluation of the Three Year "Winners" Program.* Social Research Group, School of Public Health, University of California, Berkeley.

[17]I. Rootman and J. Moser (1985) *Community Response to Alcohol-Related Problems: A World Health Organization Project Monograph.* USGPO, DHHS Publication No. (ADM) 85-1371, Washington, DC.

[18]E. G. Ritson (1985) *Community Response to Alcohol-Related Problems: Review of an International Study.* WHO, Public Health Papers No. 81, Geneva, Switzerland.

[19]L. Wallack (1984–1985) A community approach to the prevention of alcohol-related problems: the San Francisco experience. *Int. Q. Commun. Health Educ.* **5(2)**, 85–102.

[20]F. Wittman (1983) *Local Regulation of Alcohol Availability in Selected California Communities: Introduction and Summary of Findings.* Prevention Research Group, Institute of Epidemiology and Behavioral Medicine, Medical Research Institute of San Francisco, Berkeley.

[21]F. Wittman (1984) Community perspectives on the prevention of alcohol problems, in *Framework for Planning: Preventing Alcohol-Related Problems in California.* Department of Alcohol and Drug Problems, State of California Health and Welfare Agency, Sacramento.

[22]L. M. Wallack (1983) *A Community Approach to the Prevention of Alcohol-Related Problems: The San Francisco Experience.* Paper presented at the Community Prevention Research, Technical Review Conference, sponsored by the National Institute on Alcohol Abuse and Alcoholism and the National Institute of Drug Abuse, San Francisco.

[23]N. Giesbrecht and G. Conroy (1987) Options in developing community action against alcohol problems, in *Advances in Substance Abuse: Behavioral and Biological Research (Supplement 1, Control Issues in Alcohol Abuse Prevention: Strategies for State and Communities).* H. D. Holder, ed. JAI Press, Greenwich, CT, pp. 315–335.

[24]N. Giesbrecht and A. Pederson (1992) Focusing on the drinking environment or the high-risk drinker in prevention projects: limitations and opportunities, in *Community Prevention Trials for Alcohol Problems: Methodological Issues.* H. D. Holder and J. Howard, eds. Praeger, Westport, CT, pp. 97–112.

[25]S. Casswell, R. Ransom, and L. Gilmore (in press) Evaluation of a mass media campaign for the primary prevention of alcohol-related problems. *Health Promotion J.*

[26]A. Wyllie, S. Casswell, and J. Stewart (1989) The response of New Zealand boys to corporate and sponsorship alcohol advertising on television. *Br. J. Addict.* **84**, 639–646.

[27]G. Braucht and B. Braucht (1984) Prevention of problem drinking among youth: evaluation of educational strategies, in *Prevention of Alcohol Abuse.* P. Miller and T. Nirenberg, eds. Plenum, New York, pp. 253–259.

[28]R. Bangert-Drowns (1988) The effects of school-based substance abuse education: a meta-analysis. *J. Drug Educ.* **18(3)**, 243–264.

[29]W. B. Hansen (1993) School-based alcohol prevention programs. *Alcohol Health Res. World* **17(1)**, 54–60.

[30]L. Hewitt and H. Blane (1984) Prevention through mass media communication, in *Prevention of Alcohol Abuse.* P. Miller and T. Nirenberg, eds. Plenum, New York, pp. 289–323.

[31]A. Hansen (1985) Will the government's mass media campaign on drugs work? *Br. Med. J.* **290**, 1054–1055.

[32]H. Saffer and M. Grossman (1987) Beer taxes, the legal drinking age, and youth motor vehicle fatalities. *J. Legal Stud.* **16**, 351–374.

[33]P. J. Gruenewald, W. R. Ponicki, and H. D. Holder (1993) The relationship of outlet densities to alcohol consumption: a time series cross-sectional analysis. *Alcohol. Clin. Exp. Res.* **17(1)**, 38–47.

[34]P. J. Gruenewald, P. Madden, and K. Janes (1992) Alcohol availability and the formal power and resources of state alcohol beverage control agencies. *Alcohol. Clin. Exp. Res.* **16(3)**, 591–597.

[35]B. Rush, L. Gliksman, and R. Brook (1986) Alcohol availability, alcohol consumption, and alcohol-related damage. *J. Stud. Alcohol* **47**, 1–10.

[36]H. Holder and J. Blose (1987) The reduction of community alcohol problems: computer simulation experiments in three counties. *J. Stud. Alcohol* **48(2)**, 124–135.

[37]J. Blose and H. D. Holder (1987) Liquor-by-the-drink and alcohol-related traffic crashes: a natural experiment using time-series analysis. *J. Stud. Alcohol* **48(1)**, 52–60.

[38]R. Saltz (1989) Research needs and opportunities in server intervention programs. *Health Educ. Q.* **16(3)**, 429–438.

[39]A. J. McKnight (1993) Server intervention: accomplishments and needs. *Alcohol Health Res. World* **17(1)**, 76–83.

[40]M. Ashley and J. Rankin (1988) A public health approach to the prevention of alcohol-related health problems. *Annu. Rev. Public Health* **9**, 233–271.

[41]E. Single (1984) International perspectives on alcohol as a public health issue. *J. Public Health Policy* **5**, 238–256.

[42]R. Room (1984) Alcohol control and public health. *Annu. Rev. Public Health* **5**, 293–317.

[43]P. L. Zador, A. K. Lund, M. Fields, and K. Weinberg (1988) *Fatal Crash Involvement and Laws Against Alcohol-Impaired Driving.* Insurance Institute for Highway Safety, Washington, DC.

[44]R. B. Voas and J. M. Hause (1987) Deterring the drinking driver: the Stockton experience. *Accident Anal. Prev.* **19(2)**, 81–90.

[45]R. Voas, A. Rhodenizer, and C. Lynn (1985) *Evaluation of Charlottesville Checkpoint Operations.* Prepared under contract to the National Highway Traffic Safety Administration (NHTSA), #DTNH-22-83-C-05088, Washington, DC.

[46]J. Lacy, J. R. Steward, L. M. Marchetti, C. L. Popkin, P. V. Murphy, R. E. Lucke, and R. J. Jones (1986) *Enforcement and Public Information Strategies for DWI General Deterrence: Arrest Drunk Driving—The Clearwater and Largo, Florida Experience.* Technical report from the Highway Safety Research Center, University of North Carolina to U.S. Department of Transportation (DTNH22-81-C-07071), Washington, DC.

[47]R. Hingson, N. Scotch, T. Mangione, A. Myers, L. Glantz, T. Heeren, N. Mucatel, and G. Pierce (1983) Impact of legislation raising the legal drinking age in Massachusetts from 18 to 20. *Am. J. Public Health* **73**, 163–170

[48]T. Epperlein (1987) Initial deterrent effects of the crackdown on drunken drivers in the state of Arizona. *Accident Anal. Prev.* **19(4)**, 271–283.

[49]J. Mosher (1984) The impact of legal provisions on barroom behavior: toward an alcohol problem prevention strategy. *Alcohol* **1**, 205–211.

[50]R. Saltz (1987) The roles of bars and restaurants in preventing alcohol-impaired driving. *Eval. Health Professions* **10**, 5–27.

[51]M. Hennessy and R. Saltz (1989) Adjusting for multimethod bias through selection modeling. *Eval. Rev.* **13(4)**, 380–399.

[52]N. Russ and E. Geller (1987) Training bar personnel to prevent drunken driving: a field evaluation. *Am. J. Public Health* **77**, 952–954.

[53]F. Wittman (1989) Planning and programming server intervention initiatives for fraternities and sororities: experiences at a large university. *J. Primary Prev.* **9(4)**, 247–269.

[54]H. D. Holder (1989) Drinking, alcohol availability and injuries: a systems model of complex relationships, in *Drinking and Casualties: Accidents, Poisonings & Violence in an International Perspective*. N. Giesbrecht, R. Gonzalas, M. Grant, E. Osterberg, R. Room, I. Rootman, and L. Towle, eds. Associated Book Publishers, London, pp. 133–148.

[55]H. D. Holder (1993) Prevention of alcohol-related accidents in the community. *Addiction* **88(7)**, 1003–1012.

[56]J. Fell and C. Nash (1989) The nature of the alcohol problem in U.S. fatal crashes. *Health Educ. Q.* **16(3)**, 335–343.

[57]H. Richardson (1985) *Motor Vehicle Traffic Accidents as a Leading Cause of Death in the United States.* National Highway Traffic Safety Administration Research Notes No. 85-4, Washington, DC.

[58]D. Mayhew, A. Donelson, D. Beirness, and H. Simpson (1986) Youth, alcohol and relative risk of crash involvement. *Accident Anal. Prev.* **18(4)**, 273–287.

[59]P. Zador (1989) *Alcohol-Related Risk of Fatal Driver Injuries in Relation to Driver Age and Sex.* Insurance Institute for Highway Safety, Washington, DC.

[60]J. Lacy (1987) *Evaluation of North Carolina's Safe Roads Act.* Presentation to North Carolina Medical Association, Raleigh.

[61]J. Blose and H. D. Holder (1987) Public availability of distilled spirits: structural and reported consumption changes associated with liquor-by-the drink. *J. Stud. Alcohol* **48(4)**, 371–379.

[62]T. Heeren, R. Smith, S. Morelock, and R. Hingson (1985) Surrogate measures of alcohol involvement in fatal crashes: are conventional indicators adequate? *J. Safety Res.* **16**, 127–134.

[63]A. Richman (1985) Human risk factors in alcohol-related crashes. *J. Stud. Alcohol*, **Suppl. 10**, 21–31.

[64]N. Mounce, O. Pendleton, and O. Gonzales (1988) *Alcohol Involvement in Texas Driver Fatalities.* Texas Transportation Institute, Texas A&M University, College Station.

[65]R. Hingson (1987) Effects of Maine's 1981 and Massachusetts' 1982 driving-under-the-influence legislation. *Am. J. Public Health* **77(5)**, 593–597.

[66]A. Wagenaar (1986) The legal minimum drinking age in Texas: effects of an increase from 18 to 19. *J. Safety Res.* **17(4)**, 165–178.

[67]A. Wagenaar (1986) Preventing highway crashes by raising the legal minimum age for drinking: the Michigan experience six years later. *J. Safety Res.* **17(3)**, 101–109.

[68]A. Wagenaar and H. D. Holder (1991) Effects of alcoholic beverage service liability on alcohol-involved traffic crashes. *Alcohol. Clin. Exp. Res.* **15(6)**, 942–947.

[69]S. Aitken and T. Zobeck (1985) Trends in alcohol-related fatal motor-vehicle accidents for 1983. *Alcohol Health Res. World* **9**, 60–62.

[70]J. Howland and R. Hingson (1987) Alcohol as a risk factor for injuries or death due to fires or burns: review of the literature. *Public Health Rep.* **102(5)**, 475–483.

[71]R. Hingson and J. Howland (1987) Alcohol as a risk factor for injury or death resulting from accidental falls: a review of the literature. *J. Stud. Alcohol* **48(3)**, 212–219.

[72]J. Howland and R. Hingson (1989) Alcohol as a risk factor for drownings: a review of the literature. *Accident Anal. Prev.*

[73]F. J. Cairns, T. D. Koelmeyer, and W. M. I. Smeeton (1984) Deaths from drowning. *N. Zealand Med. J.* **97**, 65–67.

[74]National Transportation Safety Board (1985) *Recreational Boating Safety and Alcohol.* NTSB Report No. NTSB/55-83/02, Washington, DC.

[75]M. Mogford (1983) *An Analysis of Boating Fatalities in Ontario, 1980–1983.* Ministry of Natural Resources, Ontario.

[76]E. Press, J. Walker, and I. Crawford (1968) An interstate drowning study. *Am. J. Public Health* **58**, 2275–2289.

[77]V. Pleuckhahn (1982) Alcohol consumption and death by drowning in adults. *J. Stud. Alcohol* **43**, 445–452.

[78]C. Cherpitel (1989) A study of alcohol use and injuries among emergency room patients, in *Drinking and Casualties: Accidents, Poisonings and Violence in an International Perspective.* N. Giesbrecht et al., eds. Tavistock, London, pp. 288–299.

[79]J. W. Farquhar and S. P. Fortmann (1992) Phases for developing community trials: lessons for control of alcohol problems from research in cardiovascular disease, cancer, and adolescent health, in *Community Prevention Trials for Alcohol Problems: Methodological Issues.* H. D. Holder and J. M. Howard, eds. Praeger, Westport, CT.

[80]P. Greenwald and C. Caban (1986) A strategy for cancer prevention and control research. *Bull. World Health Organ.* **64**, 73–78.

[81]B. R. Flay (1986) Efficacy and effectiveness trials (and other phases of research) in the development of health promotion programs. *Prev. Med.* **15(5)**, 451–474.

Alcohol-Related Injuries Among Women

Mary-Ellen Fortini and Carol Lederhaus Popkin

Introduction

Although there has been a recent increase in interest of the effects of alcohol on women,[1,2] there is still a surprising paucity of research that examines alcohol-related injuries in women. Although women are often injured by intoxicated persons, the focus of this chapter is on alcohol-related injuries owing to women's drinking.

Surveillance of Alcohol Consumption and Its Consequences

Although a limited number of studies report on the presence of alcohol in injured persons, there is a lack of alcohol-related injury information by gender. Moreover, available information must be considered in light of several confounding factors. First, women drink less than men. This means there are fewer alcohol-related injuries to be reported. However, because alcohol abuse and its attendant problems are associated more frequently with men, this affects expectations, i.e., when one expects that women drink less, one is less apt to screen for alcohol involvement. For example, medical examiners generally test a lower percentage of women than men for the presence of alcohol or drugs. Failure to screen results in the underreporting of cases. Thus the possibility that there are lower testing rates for women may affect injury surveillance data, such as those used in the Fatal Accident

From: *Drug and Alcohol Abuse Reviews, Vol. 7: Alcohol, Cocaine, and Accidents*
Ed.: R. R. Watson ©1995 Humana Press Inc., Totowa, NJ

Reporting System (FARS) developed by the National Highway Traffic Safety Administration (NHTSA).

Additionally, there may be differences in the outcomes of alcohol consumption. In interviews with driving under the influence (DUI) offenders in court-sanctioned DUI programs in California,[3] a factor score variable was constructed to represent global alcohol problem severity (APS) using the Mortimer-Filkins, the Alcohol Dependence Scale, and five items from the interview protocol reflecting negative effects of alcohol (frequency of intoxication, hangovers, missing work or school, passing out, and being hospitalized). After controlling for demographic characteristics and consumption patterns, women scored higher than men on APS. Measures of quantity and frequency may not be sensitive to gender effects of alcohol consumption on alcohol problem onset.

Differential Effect of Alcohol in Women

Some laboratory studies indicate gender differences in blood alcohol concentration (BAC) levels achieved after taking a discrete dose of alcohol. Some of these are differences owing to the difference in body fat ratios between men and women. Burns and Moskowitz[4] found that, controlling for body weight, it takes 15% less alcohol for women to reach the same level of intoxication as men. Several researchers[5,6] reported that because of diminished gastric alcohol dehydrogenase, "first pass" metabolism is decreased in women and may not exist in alcoholic women. This may result in gender-related differences in BACs. However, H. Moscowitz (personal communication, May 7, 1993) reported that these differences should have only a minimal effect on women's BAC level. Some researchers suggest that variations in hormonal levels affect BAC and ethanol metabolism.[7-9] However, there are inconsistencies between the findings of various researchers.

These findings suggest that criteria currently used to identify substance abuse problems may be inappropriate for women. For example, most surveys of consumption patterns and many of the assessment instruments used to screen for substance abuse problems use five or more drinks as the benchmark for problem drinking.[10] Given the gender differences in the effects of alcohol, perhaps a better indicator of drinking problems in women would be three or four drinks.

Differences in Risk-Taking Behavior

Alcohol consumption is known to have a decremental effect on psychomotor performance. It is also associated with increases in risk-taking behavior in some. Male DUI offenders have higher scores on measures of risky driving, sensation seeking, and aggression than do women.[3] Men who drink and drive are more likely to exhibit other types of risky behavior. Several interesting studies have been made of gender differences in risk-taking behavior. Men, particularly young men, engage in more risk-taking activities,[11–13] and gender differences are reported in sensation seeking and scales of risk taking in driving.[14]

Among adolescents, women are found to have more socially acceptable attitudes toward alternatives to driving under the influence of alcohol.[15] Beck and Simmons[16] found that females were more likely to believe the consequences of drinking and driving could be serious. Werch[17] found that undergraduate females were more apt to use behavioral self-control strategies to control drinking and driving. It may be the case that women use more self-control in situations involving drinking and risk taking. A study by McMillen et al.[18] found that alcohol "enhanced" personality type, i.e., low risk takers who believed they had consumed alcohol became more careful on a simulator driving task, whereas high risk takers took more risks when they thought they had consumed alcohol.

Women also employ some behaviors that place them in positions that are less vulnerable to the consequences of drinking. They are more apt to wear their seat belts when they drink and drive.[19] They are more apt to heed warnings of others and choose to take a cab or use a designated driver if they have been drinking.[20] They apparently can become more cautious as drivers after consuming alcohol.[17]

This difference in risk-taking behavior has been underscored in a recent study by Foss et al.[19] that described results of a Minnesota Roadside Survey of drinking and occupant protection. The authors found that about one-third of late night drivers were females. Of those drivers with BACs over the legal limit, 20% were female. The peak age for intoxicated females was 25–34, compared to 21–24 for males. Interestingly, more intoxicated females were found after midnight and were coming from a friend's home (compared to a bar for males). They found that a converse relationship between BAC level and observed seat belt use in males. Women, however, were more apt to use their seat belts even when they were highly intoxicated. Safety belt use was as common among females with high BACs as those with low or no BAC. One implication of this finding is that studies based on data from fatal crashes may underestimate female drinking and driving. Because of more consistent use of safety belts, crashes involving female drivers are less likely to be fatal. Comparisons of male and female drinking drivers also show differences on personality and alcohol dependence variables. Miller et al.[21] found that females are more functional than males on measures of interpersonal competence, sensation seeking, and assaultiveness. The authors suggest that measures may be designed to identify arenas in which males are more likely to show behaviors (i.e., females may be sensation seeking but not in the areas measured with the scale).

A study of police records of arrests of women in Wichita, KS, from 1980–1984[22] profiled female arrestees as: between the ages of 20–30 (47.4%), unmarried (71.6%), and having a mean BAC of 0.18%. Most arrests had been made between midnight and 4 AM but, unlike arrests for males, were spread fairly evenly across days of the week. Recidivism rates were lower for women than men.

Other Drug Use

Most of the studies of alcohol-related injuries do not address the issue of other drug involvement. This is particularly significant because women are more frequent and chronic users of psychotropic drugs.[23] Corrigan[24] cited research that indicates a higher rate of abuse of prescription drugs and over-the-counter drugs by females than males. The role of drugs in combination with alcohol in the study of alcohol-related injuries must be taken into account when studying injuries in women.

Affect of Alcohol on Women's Ability to Perform Motor Tasks

Little information is available regarding the effect of alcohol on women's ability to perform motor tasks. Although epidemiologic studies suggest that women are at an elevated risk of crash involvement at the same BAC levels as men,[25,26] it is difficult to determine if this difference is caused by inexperience with drinking, with driving, or with a combination of both. Clearly, more research is needed in this area.

Female Tolerance to Injury

Chronic use of alcohol is important in both injury causation and outcome. It has become recognized that alcohol consumption over a prolonged period of time predisposes one to more severe injuries. Similarly, it influences the body's ability to repair itself.[27]

There is an extremely limited amount of information available on women's tolerance to injury; and even less information is available on the effect of variables that influence and perhaps may modify tolerance, such as substance abuse and restraint systems. Clearly, although women may avoid risky behaviors, they are more susceptible to injury as a result of trauma. Women in their child-bearing years are at greater risk of fatality than men in crashes of similar severity.[28]

Most gender-specific information of injury is available from motor vehicle injury literature. Apparently, fatality risk is 25% greater for females than for similarly aged males during the ages of 15–45 yr.[12] Although direct measurements are unavailable, various researchers have reported trends that indicate vulnerability of women to injury. Massie and Campbell[29] reported that between 1983 and 1990, young women experienced a decrease in relative risk of a fatal involvement and an increase in nonfatal involvements. In general, women were found to have a 26% higher injury involvement rate than men of similar age.

Popkin et al.[30] examined potential bias in police reporting of injuries. Including only accidents involving intermediate size passenger cars of model years 1980–1985 with right front occupants who were unbelted, the authors found that males were rated as not injured more often than females. However, it was not possible to say with certainty whether these differences were a result of officer-reporting bias.

The vulnerability of women is increased during their later years when smaller bones coupled with risk for osteoporosis heighten the likelihood of injuries owing to falls. Women may exacerbate this vulnerability by drinking. Prolonged consumption of alcohol takes calcium from bone, thus further weakening bone mass. Add to this the findings of Waller and colleagues[31] that indicate that alcohol potentiates the effect of injuries and one must conclude that drinking women are at risk.

Societal Protection of Women

Another factor complicating an understanding of the relationship between alcohol and injuries in women is the tendency in our society to protect women. The term "male protection syndrome" was coined to describe this process.[32] People who have a tendency to be protective are less apt to arrest women, convict women, or sentence women to penalties unless women step outside the traditional boundaries assigned to their social roles. Argeriou and Paulino[33] found support for this in their study of convicted female drunken drivers in Boston. They found that a BAC over the legal limit was a "necessary but not sufficient" cause for arrest. Convicted females, in addition to an elevated BAC, also were either verbally abusive, involved in a crash, or engaged in some other behavior that led to the arrest and conviction.

Further, police officers may be less accurate in assessing alcohol use among specific groups. It appears that officers are less accurate in assessing alcohol use by non-White females.[34] With respect to false positives, officers erroneously judged that alcohol was present in 5.48% of fatally injured non-White females, as contrasted to 2.5% of White females. The officer in this small number of cases correctly indicated drinking in 75% of the cases involving White females, but only 50% of the cases involving non-White females.

Given the aforementioned factors, let us examine the involvement of alcohol in injuries. Data on the prevalence of drinking by women are available from several sources: national surveys, roadside surveys on drinking and driving, reports of hospital admissions for alcohol and substance abuse treatment, and morbidity and mortality studies.

There are some inconsistencies in the reporting of changes in alcohol consumption by women. First, it is well documented that women drink less than men. Several surveys report that women are not experiencing substantial changes in heavy drinking and alcoholism.[35,36] However, although as a group there have not been substantial increases in alcohol problems/alcoholism, among certain subgroups there appear to be increases in drinking behavior. For example, Wilsnack and Beckman[36] found that unmarried women cohabitating following high school were among the subgroups of women most likely to be drinkers and most likely to be moderate to heavy drinkers. Fillmore[37] found an increase in heavy drinking among 21–29-yr old females.

Alcohol-Related Injuries Involving Women

Motor Vehicle Injuries

Although there have been few studies that directly examine alcohol-related vehicular injuries of women, accident report data for both males and females are available from FARS, driver records, and emergency rooms. Women traditionally drive fewer miles than men and often drive at times that represent lower risk of crash involvement.[38] In the United States, the proportion of drivers who are women has been increasing steadily, particularly among older aged women.

In the United States, females account for 48.6% of all drivers, 35.2% of all travel time, 37.9% of all police-reported crashes, and 23.9% of all fatal crashes.[39] Females show slightly higher crash involvement rates than males when estimates of driving exposure (i.e., miles driven) are taken into account. However, as Popkin[40] discussed, the demand of the driving task is not available in current exposure data. Males traditionally drive during periods of higher risk, in inclement weather, and at night. Women have higher crash involvement rates and higher injury rates per miles driven than men after the age of 30.[29]

Fatal Injuries

The most complete data are maintained on fatally injured drivers. Involvement in a fatal crash may be affected by several factors, including crash worthiness of the car, occupant restraint use, and, of course, alcohol use. The most comprehensive data available on the involvement of alcohol in motor vehicle injuries are provided by the FARS. Alcohol-related crashes account for 50–55% of all crashes.[41]

It is known that the relative risk of motor vehicle injury increases as BAC increases for both males and females.[26] However, the relative risk lines are different with risk for females. FARS estimates show that from 1982–1992, alcohol-related fatal crash involvement rates per 100,000 licensed drivers declined 21% for men but only 16% for women. Fell,[41] using information obtained from FARS, reported on alcohol involvement in fatal crashes and found that from 1982–1985, overall, female involvement rate decreased almost as much as involvement rates for men, but that rates for 21–24-yr-old females did not change during that 4-yr period and might even have increased. Also, the younger group's involvement in single vehicle nighttime crashes was almost as high as that for male drivers during the hours of midnight to 6 AM. (Single vehicle nighttime crashes are often used as a surrogate measure for alcohol involvement because they cannot be influenced by officer bias in labeling a crash as alcohol-related.)

Although alcohol involvement in fatal crashes decreased dramatically from 1982–1985 for both genders and most age groups, there was no change for females ages 21–24. For this age group of women, alcohol consumption is also relatively high. It is interesting to note that although alcohol involvement did decrease for both genders, female involvement did not decrease as much as male involvement. Although the rate of intoxication among male drivers involved in fatal crashes is much higher than that for females between 6 PM and midnight, the rates of males and females are very close between the hours of midnight and 6 AM.

Popkin and Council[34] examined trends in alcohol-related drinking behavior in North Carolina from 1974–1988 and reported that although there were substantial declines for males after passage of alcohol-related driving legislation, similar declines were not observed in alcohol-related crash trends of White and non-White females. They report that with respect to females, fatal crash-related findings indicate that crashes involving young White females and older non-White females were more likely to involve alcohol use. Specifically, they found that 35% of fatally injured White females ages 21–24 had mean BACs greater than or equal to 0.10, as contrasted to only 14% of their non-White female counterparts. In the groups of fatally injured drivers 55+, the findings were reversed, with 36% of non-White female drivers showing BACs over 0.10 vs only 8% of White female drivers. The BAC levels of fatally injured women drivers is 0.085 for 21–24-yr-old White women and 0.030 for non-White women of the same age. For 55+, the mean BAC level for White female fatally injured drivers was 0.015 as compared to 0.065 for non-White females.

Nonfatal Injuries

Epidemiologic studies of alcohol involvement in nonfatal motor vehicle crashes is limited. McLellan et al.[42] undertook a 3-yr study of alcohol involvement in nonfatally injured drivers admitted to a trauma center in Canada. Female patients represented 23.4% of the drivers and 16.3% of those with a positive alcohol concentration.

A series of studies by Popkin and colleagues in North Carolina indicated increasing involvement in drinking and driving for women relative to men among younger age groups.[43] The North Carolina study compared young (under 36) women to young men on rates of alcohol-related driving activity, alcohol-related crashes, crash surrogates, and single vehicle nighttime crashes, from the mid-1970s to the mid-1980s. When alcohol-related crashes and single vehicle nighttime crashes were examined separately by age and gender, all subcategories of males experienced declines in both directly identified alcohol-related crashes and in single vehicle nighttime crashes; however, all but one age category of females experienced an increase in involvement. Among females ages 21–24, involvement rates for alcohol-related crashes increased by 93%, as compared to a 7% decline for male counterparts. These patterns generally supported increased drinking and driving as well as increased alcohol-related crash experiences among young women, an increase that was not explained entirely by overall increased driving exposure.

Other Alcohol-Related Injuries/Fatalities

Most of the studies employ coroner reports and/or emergency room records. Although these methods yield important information regarding alcohol involvement at the time of the injury or death, there are several limitations to these studies. First, not all victims are tested for blood alcohol. As mentioned earlier, the factors that determine whether or not a victim will be tested may be systematically biased.

Using data from medical examiners from Oklahoma, Goodman and colleagues[44] found that the rate of testing for blood alcohol varied by type of death: 90% of homicide victims, 73% of suicide victims, and 66% of unintentional fatal injuries (all fatal injuries other than homicide or suicide) were tested for blood alcohol level (for persons who died on the same day they were injured). Forty-nine percent of the unintentional injuries were alcohol-related; 38% with alcohol levels over 0.10%. For homicide victims, 52% were alcohol positive, 34% with levels over 0.10%. For suicide victims, 40% were alcohol-related, 24% over the limit of 0.10%.

Goodman et al.[44] also reported that there were gender differences related to race/culture. Among Hispanic, Black, and White populations, male victims were more likely than females to test positive for alcohol. For Native Americans, however, 80% of the unintentional injury deaths were alcohol positive regardless of gender. About 60% of the females and 70% of the males had blood alcohol levels over 0.10%. There were some differences in the Native American population related to tribal memberships. Because of the differences in testing in each county and the fact that the sample is only from Oklahoma, there is some question as to the generalizability of the results. It is, however, one of the few studies that examines the role of alcohol in fatal injuries that accounts for gender and ethnic differences.

There are little data available on the incidence of alcohol-related injuries in women among hospitalized patients. Reports from a Level I trauma center,[45] that routinely conducts alcohol screens on patients admitted for trauma-related injuries, provides information on 1467 women and 3779 men. BACs were positive in 22.9% of women and 40.3% of men. The mean BAC level was 154 mg/dL for women and 166 mg/dL for men. Seventy-four percent of women with a positive BAC were at or above the *per se* legal limit (0.10%), compared with 79% for males.

Thirty-eight percent of women, as contrasted to 49% of men, involved in motor vehicle crashes had positive BACs. In assault cases, 23% of women and 45% of men had positive BACs. Grouping other injury mishaps together, including burns, falls, and so on, 16% of women as compared with 35% of men had positive BACs.

Using national hospital discharge survey data, Towle et al.[46] examined proportionate morbidity for injuries and accidents coded in alcohol-related charges for males and females separately. For both injuries and accidents, proportionate morbidity appears to be slightly greater for females than for males, with the differences being larger for the accident diagnosis. They found that females with chronic alcohol-related diagnoses are more likely than males to have mention of an accident on their discharge record. This may be because females are more likely to report poor driving performance than males. Injury rates and accident rates for females as well as males indicate an upward trend during 1979–1985.

In a series of emergency room studies, Cherpitel and colleagues[47-50] reported on alcohol- and violence-related injuries. Among all males and females above the age of 30, those with violence-related injuries were more likely than those with other injuries to have positive breathalyzer readings and to report drinking prior to the event.

A small number of studies have been conducted to examine alcohol-related workplace injuries. In a study of occupationally related deaths in Harris County, TX,[51] autopsies were performed on 95% of the 207 deaths in 1984 and 1985. BACs were obtained for 88% of those autopsied. Thirteen percent were positive for alcohol, with 9% over 0.10%. Only 14 of the deaths were women and none tested were positive for alcohol.

Alcohol-Related Mortality

According to Herd,[52] between 1950 and 1973 there have been dramatic increases in the age-adjusted death rates for liver cirrhosis among women, including non-Whites. Williams et al.[53] reported that cirrhosis mortality for non-White females, although similar to those of White females from 1945–1952, had increased to almost twice the rate for White females in 1973, and has remained at about twice the rate.

Death certificates and autopsy information have provided data for studies on alcohol-related injuries. For example, Pignon[54] found that 9% of all deaths in France in 1985 were attributable to alcohol, 6% for males and 3% for females. According to the 1987 Stockholm death certificates, 9.2% of males and 11.2% of females reported alcohol (either alcoholism, intoxication, pancreatitis, or cirrhosis) as the cause of death.[55] A reevaluation of additional information available regarding the death (e.g., autopsy information, police records, and information about earlier convictions) led to the reclassification of cause of death to include alcohol so that 57.5% of males and 32.2% of females included alcohol involvement. This reclassification was most marked for those deaths that listed injury as the cause of death.

Similarly, Stinson and colleagues[56] showed that when alcohol-attributable fractions (AAFs) were applied to the total number of deaths for each underlying cause, alcohol-related mortality was the fourth leading cause of death in the United States for all races and both sexes from 1979–1989. Examination by gender showed that for Black women, alcohol-related mortality was the fourth leading cause and for White females the sixth.

In a study by Sutocky and colleagues,[57] alcohol-related mortality, rates and years of potential life lost were calculated using California mortality data from 1989. Over 6% of all deaths in California were alcohol related. Of all alcohol-related deaths, women accounted for 31.8%. Alcohol-related deaths accounted for 4.1% of all women's deaths (compared to 8% of male deaths). Motor vehicle accidents accounted for the largest contributor to women's alcohol-related mortality (15.7%, followed by cerebrovascular diseases (14.6%) and alcoholic cirrhosis of the liver (10.1%). For intentional injuries, the estimated mortality rate for women was 12.2% (compared to 21.9% for men). For unintentional injuries (including motor vehicle,

Table 1
Estimated Alcohol-Related Mortality (ARM)
and Mortality Rates for Injuries California, 1989[a]

Diagnosis	AAF[b]	Male		Female	
		ARM	Rate	ARM	Rate
Unintentional injuries					
Motor vehicle accidents	0.42	1698	11.85	663	4.50
Other road vehicle accidents	0.20	5	0.03	1	0.01
Water transport accidents	0.20	9	0.06	2	0.01
Air/space transport accidents	0.16	19	0.13	4	0.03
Alcohol poisonings	1.00	25	0.23	4	0.03
Accidental falls	0.35	214	1.96	142	1.24
Accidents caused by fires	0.45	72	0.50	54	0.37
Accidental drownings	0.38	134	0.94	44	0.30
Other injuries	0.25	187	1.71	64	0.56
Intentional injuries					
Suicide	0.28	814	7.45	252	2.20
Homicide	0.46	1166	10.67	261	2.28

[a]Excerpted from Sutocky et al. (1993).[57]
[b]Alcohol attributable factor.

other road vehicle, water transport, air/space transport accidents, poisonings, falls, fires, drownings, and other injuries) the estimated mortality rate for females was 23.2% (compared to 26.1% for males). Table 1 shows the estimated alcohol-related mortality and mortality rates.

Alcohol-related years of potential life lost (YPLL) to age 65 and to life expectancy were calculated. Regardless of gender, alcohol-related injury deaths (both intentional and unintentional) accounted for a mean of almost 40 YPLL to life expectancy. The YPLL to age 65 for injury deaths was approx 23 yr for females and 28 yr for males. The classification as alcohol-related death is limited in that it is based solely on mortality data using "underlying cause of death." Since it is unclear for some of the underlying causes whether alcohol was involved, it is likely that alcohol-related deaths are underestimated. There are little data available on the incidence of alcohol-related injuries in women among hospital patients. Data perhaps exist, but have not been analyzed and described in the research literature.

Falls

Falls comprise the second leading cause of unintentional injuries. Although alcohol is purported to be involved in falls, there is little epidemiological research examining alcohol involvement in falls and almost none examines the use of alcohol by women. Murphy and Moore[58] examined falls on escalators and found that alcohol was a factor in 74% of the male cases but only 6% of the female cases.

Poisoning

The third leading cause of unintentional injury deaths are poisonings. Twenty-seven percent of deaths by poisoning involve women.[59] However, few poisonings are directly attributable to the ingestion of alcohol. Additional research is needed on the use of alcohol as a contributing factor in these injuries rather than the injury-inducing substance.

Drowning/Aquatic Activities

Drownings are the fifth most common cause of death in the United States. Howland et al.[60] reviewed the literature on alcohol-related drowning deaths and reported that these studies indicate that 25–50% of drownings involve alcohol. They felt there was insufficient information available to directly attribute cause of death to alcohol. According to Howland et al.[61] the ratio of male:female drownings is 12:1 for drownings associated with a boat and 5:1 for other drownings. It is interesting to note that they found that gender differences in drowning rates did not change with age.

Howland et al.[60] conducted a telephone survey of 2706 persons over the age of 16 from a random sample of US households. Of respondents, 74% of males and 66% of females reported alcohol use. Of alcohol users, 52% of males and 34% of females had consumed alcohol on at least one occasion while participating in an aquatic activity. Men reported drinking a mean of 4.5 alcoholic beverages and women an average of 2.9. It should be noted that the mean number of drinks consumed on the last day on or near the water was five for females ages 16–20 and four for females ages 21–25. The male:female ratio of drowning rates was 14:1 in the United States.

Patteta and Biddinger[62] examined the characteristics of drowning deaths in North Carolina and found that the overall rate per 100,000 was 3.2 with 0.7 deaths per 100,000 residents for White females and 1.2 for non-White females. Females were more apt to die while bathing or secondary to a motor vehicle crash and most of these were passengers in vehicles. Forty-one percent of White females 15 yr and above who drowned had some alcohol in their bodies and 24% of them had BAC levels at or above 0.10%. Among non-White females, 28% had alcohol in their systems at the time of death and 19% of them had BAC levels at or above 0.10%.

Wintemute et al.[63] examined selected cases from coroner reports of drowning victims in Sacramento, CA, from 1974–1985. They found that 41% of drownings were alcohol related. Furthermore, they found that alco-

Table 2
North Carolina Resident Suicides
by Race, Sex, Age Group, Method, and Alcohol Level, 1985–1989[a]

	Total suicides	Firearm-related suicides	Tested for alcohol	BAC ≥.10
White male				
Age 0–64	2168	1628 (75.1%)	1987	603 (30.3%)
Age 65+	605	524 (86.6%)	533	46 (8.6%)
White female				
Age 0–64	627	330 (52.6%)	575	83 (14.4%)
Age 65+	129	58 (45.0%)	111	7 (6.3%)
Non-White male				
Age 0–64	333	249 (74.8%)	315	65 (20.6%)
Age 65+	48	40 (83.3%)	39	3 (7.7%)
Non-White female				
Age 0–64	75	35 (46.7%)	58	13 (22.4%)
Age 65+	14	6 (42.9%)	11	0 (0.0%)

[a]Unpublished research, Michael Patetta, Department of Environment, Health and Natural Resources, Injury Control, 1993.

hol was associated with drowning in 59% of drownings involving males and 40% among females. A BAC ≥100 mg/dL was obtained in 40% of male and 27% of female drownings. Branch et al.[64] examined spinal injuries resulting from diving accidents and found that those who were injured were four times more likely to have used alcohol than were control cases.

Suicide and Self-Destructive Behaviors

In a study of suicide risk among women with alcohol problems, Gomberg[23] matched groups of alcoholic and nonalcoholic women on age and socioeconomic status of family of origin. She reported that 40% of the alcoholics had made suicide attempts, compared to 8.8% of the nonalcoholics. Younger alcoholics were twice as likely as alcoholics over 40 to attempt suicide. In a review of the literature on alcohol-related self-destructive behaviors, Ferrence[65] concluded that female alcoholics are at a greater risk of suicide than other females but that this difference is significantly smaller between male alcoholics and other men.

In an unpublished study of suicide among North Carolina residents from 1985–1989, the total number of deaths classified as suicides amid the proportion of decedents with BACs at or above 0.10 were examined (*see* Table 2). Older persons were less likely to have high BACs than younger persons. Thirty percent of White males under 65 yr of age had high BAC levels, compared to 21% of non-White males. Among females under 65 yr, 14% of Whites and 22% of non-Whites had BAC levels at or above 0.10%. For females age 65 or older, the rates were 6 and 0% for Whites and non-Whites, respectively.

Homicide

Studies indicate that alcohol is used by both victim and perpetrator in nearly two-thirds of the cases. Parker,[66] in a cross-cultural study on the effects of alcohol and divorce on homicide victimization, reported that although alcohol consumption and drinking style (on the national level) did not directly affect homicide victimization, there was an interaction with the gender of the victim. The relationship between "mixed" drinking style (those countries, including the United States, in which alcohol has an ambivalent place in the social and cultural framework) and divorce impacted on the rate of female victimization but not on male victimization.

Goodman et al.[67] examined BACs of 4000 Los Angeles homicide victims from 1970–1979 and found that 26% of female victims had detectable levels of alcohol in their blood (51% of males victims did). Hamilton and Collins[68] reviewed studies of husband to wife domestic violence. The most common pattern was for both parties to have been drinking. Situations in which only the victim had been drinking occurred about 13% of the time. As Collins and Messerschmidt[69] suggested, people under the influence of alcohol may have severely diminished capability of accurately assessing risk.

Summary

Data sources available to study alcohol-related injuries in women include police records of motor vehicle crashes, emergency department records, and morbidity and mortality data. However, with few exceptions, gender-specific research on the effect of alcohol on injury causation and potentiation is limited. Undoubtedly there are large data sets that contain gender-specific injury information that have been aggregated for methodological reasons. Researchers may wish to disaggregate these to examine gender differences and trends more closely. If women are impaired at lower BAC levels, different ranges of BAC should be examined when considering gender-related differences in alcohol-related injuries. For example, perhaps researchers could examine gender differences in injury at different BAC levels.

The limited data that are available suggest complex sets of issues that warrant further research. These include the effect of alcohol on an individual's ability to avoid dangerous situations. For example, in studies of alcohol's involvement in drownings, a substantial number of women report having consumed alcohol while engaged in aquatic activities. Yet the ratio of male:female deaths was 14:1. How are these differences explained? Another area of research might be the examination of the effect of alcohol in potentiating injury. Are women more vulnerable to injury because they have smaller bones?

In our review of the literature we found that women have fewer injuries than men and also that women consume smaller quantities of alcohol. The fact that women drink less and that they are less risk taking in their behavior would suggest that fewer of them are candidates for alcohol-related injuries. There are some indications that certain subpopulations of women are increasing their consumption of alcohol and also that women are increasing some risk-taking behaviors. The facts intuitively suggest that a greater understanding is needed of the relative risk of women to certain injuries. However, to better understand the role of alcohol in injuries to women, BACs must be obtained more regularly and the biases inherent in the research must be addressed.

References

[1]S. B. Blume (1986) Women and alcohol: a review. *JAMA* **256,** 1467–1470.

[2]P. Roman (1988) *Women and Alcohol Use: A Review of the Research Literature.* DHHS Publication No. (ADM) 88–1574, US Department of Health and Human Services, Washington, DC.

[3]B. J. Anderson, M. W. Perrine, A. R. Meyers, and M. E. Fortini (1992) Male and female DUI offenders: a comparison of psychosocial characteristics, in *Proceedings of the International Conference on Alcohol, Drugs, and Traffic Safety, T92.* H.-D. Utzelmann, G. Berghaus, and G. Kroj, eds. Verlag TÜV Rheinland, Cologne, Germany, pp. 1110–1116.

[4]M. Burns and H. Moskowitz (1980) *Methods for Estimating Expected Blood Alcohol Concentration.* Southern California Research Institute (National Traffic Information System: DOT HS-805-563), Los Angeles.

[5]M. Frezza, C. DiPadova, G. Pozzato, M. Terpin, E. Baraona, and C. S. Lieber (1990) High blood levels in women: the role of decreased gastric alcohol dehydrogenase activity and first-pass metabolism. *N. Engl. J. Med.* **322,** 95–99.

[6]R. J. Julkunen, L. Tannenbaum, E. Baraona, and C. S. Lieber (1985) First pass metabolism of ethanol: an important determinant of blood levels after alcohol consumption. *Alcohol* **2,** 437–441.

[7]B. M. Jones and M. K. Jones (1976) Women and alcohol: intoxication, metabolism, and the menstrual cycle, in *Alcoholism Problems in Women and Children.* M. Greenblatt and M. Shuckit, eds. Grune and Stratton, New York, pp. 103–136.

[8]W. M. Hayes, P. E. Nathan, H. W. Heermans, and W. Frankenstein (1984) Menstrual cycle tolerance and blood level discrimination. *Addict. Behav.* **9,** 67–77.

[9]P. S. Kegg and A. R. Zeiner (1980) Birth control pill effects on ethanol pharmokinetics, acetaldehyde and cardiovascular measures in Caucasian females. *Psychophysiology* **17**, 94. (abstract)

[10]C. L. Popkin, C. K. Kannenberg, J. L. Lacey, and P. F. Waller (1988) *Assessment of Classification Instruments Designed to Detect Alcohol Abuse.* National Highway Traffic Safety Administration. DOT HS 807475, Washington, DC.

[11]D. M. Donovan and G. A. Marlatt (1982) Personality subtypes among driving-while-intoxicated offenses: relationship to drinking behavior and driving risk. *J. Consult. Clin. Psychol.* **50**, 241–249.

[12]L. Evans (1991) *Traffic Safety and the Driver.* Van Reinhold, New York.

[13]R. J. Wilson (1991) Subtypes of DUIs and high risk drivers: implications for differential intervention. *Alcohol, Drugs, Driving* **7**, 1–12.

[14]A. Furnham and J. Saipe (1993) Personality correlates of convicted drivers. *Personality Diff.* **14**, 329–336.

[15]J. Farrow and P. Brissing (1990) Risk for DWI: a new look at gender differences in drinking and driving influences, experiences, and attitudes among adolescent drivers. *Health Educ. Q.* **17**, 213–221.

[16]K. H. Beck and T. G. Simmons (1987) Adolescent gender differences in alcohol beliefs and behaviors. *J. Alcohol Drug Educ.* **33**, 311–344.

[17]C. E. Werch (1990) Behavioral self-control strategies for deliberately limiting drinking among college students. *Addict. Behav.* **15**, 119–128.

[18]D. L. McMillen, S. Smith, and E. N. Wells-Parker (1989) The effects of alcohol, expectancy, and sensation-seeking on driving risk taking. *Addict. Behav.* **14**, 477–483.

[19]R. D. Foss, R. B. Voas, D. J. Beirness, and A. C. Wolf (1990) *Minnesota Roadside Survey of Drinking and Driving 1990. Final Report.* Department of Public Safety, St. Paul.

[20]J. H. Pandiani and R. J. McGrath (1986) Attempts to dissuade drinkers from driving: the effect of driver characteristics. *J. Drug Educ.* **16**, 341–348.

[21]B. A. Miller, T. H. Nochajski, and W. F. Wieczorek (1992) *Personality and Behavioral Characteristics of Female and Male Drinking Drivers.* Research Society on Alcohol Annual meeting.

[22]E. R. Shore, M. L. McCoy, L. A. Toonen, and E. J. Kuntz (1988) Arrests of women for driving under the influence. *J. Stud. Alcohol* **49**, 7–10.

[23]E. S. L. Gomberg (1989) Suicide risk among women with alcohol problems. *Am. J. Public Health* **79**, 1363–1365.

[24]E. M. Corrigan (1985) Gender differences in alcohol and other drug use. *Addict. Behav.* **10**, 313–317.

[25]M. M. Hyman (1968) The social characteristics of persons arrested while intoxicated. *Q. J. Stud. Alcohol* **4**, 138–177.

[26]P. L. Zador (1991) Alcohol related relative risk of fatal driver injuries in relation to driver age and sex. *J. Stud. Alcohol* **52**, 302–310.

[27]*Injury in America. A Continuing Public Health Problem* (1985) National Academy Press, Washington, DC.

[28]L. Evans (1988) Risk of fatality from physical trauma versus sex and age. *J. Trauma* **28**, 368–378.

[29]D. L. Massie and K. L. Campbell (1993) *Analysis of Accident Rates by Age, Gender and Time of Day Based on the 1990 Nationwide Transportation Survey.* University of Michigan Transportation Research Institute, Ann Arbor.

[30]C. L. Popkin, B. J. Campbell, A. R. Hansen, and J. R. Stewart (1991) *Analysis of the Accuracy of the Existing KABCO Injury Scale.* University of North Carolina Report Number PR180, University of North Carolina Highway Safety Research Center, Chapel Hill.

[31]P. F. Waller, F. Hansen, J. R. Stewart, C. L. Popkin, and E. Rodgman (1987) The potentiating effects of alcohol on injury. *JAMA* **256**, 1461–1466.

[32]P. Scoles and E. W. Fine (1981) Some considerations of alcohol use and drinking driving behavior in women. *Focus Women* **2**, 133–144.

[33]M. Argeriou and D. Paulino (1976) Women arrested for drunken driving in Boston: social characteristics and circumstances of arrest. *J. Stud. Alcohol* **37**, 648–658.

[34]C. L. Popkin and F. M. Council (1993) A comparison of alcohol-related driving behavior of white and non-white North Carolina drivers. *Accident Anal. Prev.* **25**, 355–364.

[35]D. S. Haskin, B. Grant, and T. C. Harford (1990) Male and female differences in liver cirrhosis mortality in the United States, 1961–1985. *J. Stud. Alcohol* **51**, 123–129.

[36]S. C. Wilsnack and L. J. Beckman, eds. (1984) *Alcohol Problems in Women: Antecedents, Consequences, and Interventions.* Guilford, New York.

[37]K. M. Fillmore (1984) "When angels fall": women's drinking as cultural preoccupation and as reality, in *Alcohol Problems in Women.* S. C. Wilsnack and L. J. Beckman, eds. Guilford, New York, pp. 7–36.

[38]C. L. Popkin, L. C. Rudisill, P. F. Waller, and S. B. Geissinger (1988) Female drinking and driving: recent trends in North Carolina. *Accident Anal. Prev.* **20**, 219–225.

[39]E. C. Cerrelli (1992) *Crash Data and Rates for Age-Sex Groups of Drivers, 1990.* National Highway Traffic Safety Administration Department of Transportation Research Note, Washington, DC.

[40]C. L. Popkin (1993) A consideration of factors influencing drinking and driving by women. *Alcohol, Drugs, Driving* **9**, 197–210.

[41]J. C. Fell (1987) *Alcohol Involvement Rates in Fatal Crashes: A Focus on Young Drivers and Female Drivers.* National Highway Traffic Safety Administration Technical Report, DOT HS 807 184, Washington, DC.

[42]B. A. McLellan, E. Vingilis, C. B. Liban, and G. Stoduto (1990) Blood alcohol testing of motor vehicle crash victims at a regional trauma unit. *J. Trauma* **30**, 418–421.

[43]C. L. Popkin (1991) Drinking and driving by young females. *Accident Anal. Prev.* **23**, 37–44.

[44]R. A. Goodman, G. R. Istre, F. B. Jordan, J. L. Herndon, and J. Kelaghan (1991) Alcohol and fatal injuries in Oklahoma. *J. Stud. Alcohol* **52**, 156–161.

[45]C. A. Soderstrom and P. Dischinger (1993) (personal communication) Preliminary findings of patients admitted to R. Adams Cowley Shock Trauma Center, Baltimore, MD

[46]L. H. Towle, F. S. Stinson, and M. Dufour (1988) Assessment of the potential for surveillance of alcohol-related casualties using national hospital discharge survey data. *Public Health Rep.* **103**, 597–605.

[47]C. J. S. Cherpitel (1989) Breath analysis and self-reports as measures of alcohol related emergency room admissions. *J. Stud. Alcohol* **50**, 155–161.

[48]C. J. S. Cherpitel and H. Rosovsky (1990) Alcohol consumption and casualties: a comparison of emergency room populations in the United States and Mexico. *J. Stud. Alcohol* **51**, 319–326.

[49]C. J. Cherpitel (1993) Alcohol and violence-related injuries: an emergency room study. *Addiction* **88**, 79–88.

[50]C. J. Cherpitel, A. Pares, and J. Rodes (1993) Prediction of alcohol-related casualties in the emergency room: a U.S.–Spain comparison. *J. Stud. Alcohol* **54,** 308–314.

[51]R. J. Lewis and S. P. Cooper (1989) Alcohol, other drugs, and fatal work-related injuries. *J. Occupat. Med.* **31,** 23–28.

[52]D. Herd (1985) The epidemiology of drinking patterns and alcohol related problems among U.S. Blacks, in *Alcohol Use Among U.S. Ethnic Minorities.* National Institute on Alcohol Abuse and Alcoholism, Research Monograph 18, Washington, DC.

[53]G. D. Williams, B. F. Grant, F. S. Stinson, T. S. Zobeck, S. A. Aitken, and J. Noble (1988) Trends in alcohol related morbidity and mortality. *Public Health Rep.* **103,** 592–597.

[54]J. P. Pignon and C. Hill (1991) Nombre de deces attributables à l'alcool, en France, en 1985 (Estimation of alcohol-related deaths in France, 1985). *Gastroenterol. Clin. Biol.* **15,** 51–56.

[55]A. Romelsjo, G. Karlsson, L. Henningsohn, and S. W. Jakobsson (1993) The prevalence of alcohol-related mortality in both sexes: variation between indicators, Stockholm, 1987. *Am. J. Public Health* **83,** 838–844.

[56]F. S. Stinson, M. C. Dufour, R. A. Steffens, and S. F. DeBakey (1993) Alcohol-related mortality in the United States. *Alcohol Health Res. World* **17,** 251–260.

[57]J. W. Sutocky, J. M. Shultz, and K. W. Kizer (1993) Alcohol-related mortality in California, 1980–1989. *Am. J. Public Health* **83,** 817–823.

[58]J. P. Murphy and F. P. Moore (1992) Escalator injuries. *Injury* **29,** 336–338.

[59]National Safety Council (1992) *Accident Facts, 1992 Edition.* Author, Itasca, IL.

[60]J. Howland, R. Hingson, T. Heeren, S. Vak, and T. Mangione (1993) Alcohol use and aquatic activities—United States, 1991. *MMWR* **42,** 675–683.

[61]J. Howland, R. Hingson, A. Lenison, M. Winter, and T. Mangione (1990) Alcohol use and aquatic activities—Massachusetts, 1988. *MMWR* **39,** 332–334.

[62]M. J. Patetta and P. W. Biddinger (1988) Characteristics of drowning deaths in North Carolina. *Public Health Rep.* **103,** 406–411.

[63]G. J. Wintemute, S. P. Teret, J. F. Kraus, and M. Wright (1990) Alcohol and drowning: an analysis of contributing factors and a discussion of criteria for case selection. *Accident Anal. Prev.* **22,** 291–296.

[64]C. M. Branch, J. E. Sniezek, R. W. Sattin, and I. R. Mirkin (1991) Water recreation-related spinal injuries: risk factors in natural bodies of water. *Accident Anal. Prev.* **23,** 13–17.

[65]R. G. Ferrence (1989) Sex differences in alcohol-related casualties: the case of self-destructive behavior, in *Accidents, Poisonings, and Violence in an International Perspective.* N. Giesbrecht, R. Gonzalez, M. Grant, E. Osterberg, R. Room, I. Rootman, and L. Towle, eds. Routledge, New York, pp. 343–355.

[66]R. N. Parker (1993) *Alcohol, Homicide, and Cultural Context: A Cross National Analysis of Gender Specific Homicide Victimization.* Manuscript submitted.

[67]R. A. Goodman, J. A. Mercy, F. Loya, M. I. Rosenberg, J. C. Smith, N. H. Allen, L. Vargas, and R. Kolts (1986) Alcohol use and interpersonal violence: alcohol detected in homicide victims. *Am. J. Public Health* **76,** 144–149.

[68]C. J. Hamilton and J. J. Collins (1981) The role of alcohol in wife beating and child abuse, in *Drinking and Crime: Perspectives on the Relationship Between Alcohol Consumption and Criminal Behavior.* J J. Collins, ed. Guilford, New York, pp. 253–287.

[69]J. J. Collins and P. M. Messerschmidt (1993) Epidemiology of alcohol-related violence. *Alcohol Health Res. World* **17,** 93–100.

Index